WHAT IS A
Defibrillator?

A CARDIOLOGIST'S GUIDE FOR PATIENTS AND CARE PROVIDERS

Dr. Jeffrey L. Williams

ISBN: 1514725703
ISBN 13: 9781514725702
Library of Congress Control Number: 2015902615
CreateSpace Independent Publishing Platform
North Charleston, South Carolina

To my wife and three great kids without whose never-failing patience and sheer bribery (on my part) for the time to spend writing, I would have never completed this book.

To my patients for, well...tolerating me.

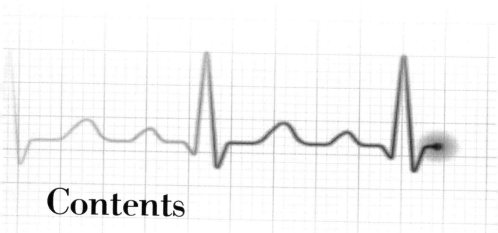

Contents

List of Figures

List of Tables

Introduction

The hectic pace at which today's doctors conduct their practices has shortchanged the information-sharing process for patients undergoing device (pacemaker or defibrillator) implantation. Patients and their families are often unaware of many critical issues involved in defibrillator implantation. Any surgery entails risks that are particular for each procedure and patient, although defibrillator implantation per se can usually be performed with minimal risks. I have found it increasingly difficult to provide a complete consultation, physical exam, and discussion about the risks, benefits, and alternatives of defibrillator implantation in a typical forty-five-minute session. Since starting the Heart Rhythm Center in 2008, I have developed several iterations of written and online patient-education materials to complement our office discussions. This book serves as a comprehensive summary of the steps involved with defibrillator implantation, from the initial evaluation and implantation procedure to the possible postoperative complications and required long-term follow-up care for patients and their caregivers (both professional and lay-people alike). Furthermore, many of my patients (young and old) rely upon their spouses and families for help with the decision-making process and long-term care of their devices. This book serves as a thorough means to ensure that all family members understand the roles, risks, and required follow-up for defibrillator patients.

Over 300,000 patients undergo defibrillator implantation in the world each year; the United States alone accounts for around 130,000 defibrillator implants annually (Mond and Proclemer 2011). There are reports of defibrillator-implant complications; generally they are outcomes and incident-complication rates reported by clinical trials. There are fewer reports of complication rates in the extreme elderly (with a persistent exclusion of elderly patients from ongoing clinical trials; Cherubini et al. 2011).

This is the first and only book dedicated solely to patients, families, and their (other) care providers as a comprehensive review of the "what, why, and how" of defibrillator implantation. As our patients become more and more invested in decisions that affect their health care, they need more detailed information in order to make comprehensive assessments before proceeding with any surgical procedures. This book can be part of the informed-consent process, because it covers more thoroughly the entire defibrillator-implantation process than can be presented in a single office visit or even multiple visits. Chapters 1, 2, and 3 offer very detailed discussions about heart function and reasons for defibrillator implantation—I've tried not to over-whelm the reader but felt that I needed to include advanced information for readers that would like this level of detail. Particular emphasis will be placed on the complications that can occur during and after defibrillator implantation and on ways to assess a particular defibrillator implanter's odds of a successful operation. If you don't understand some of the words in this text, there is a full glossary at the end of the book. Ultimately, patients who are concerned that they may need defibrillators will find this book a use-ful summary of the complete evaluation that is performed to see if a defibrillator may be of benefit. One of the most important things to remember is that most defibrillators are pacemakers, but pacemakers are *not* defibrillators.

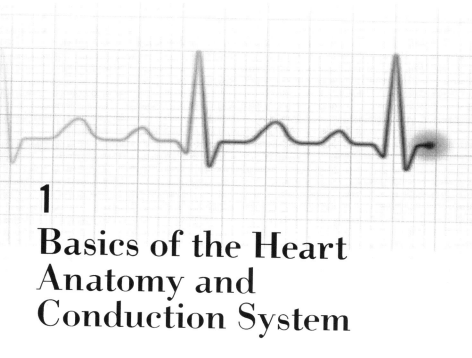

1
Basics of the Heart Anatomy and Conduction System

Blood flow through the heart. Figure 1 depicts the basic structure of the heart. Blood returns from the body and enters the right atrium. The blood leaves the right atrium through the tricuspid valve and enters the right ventricle. The right ventricle then pumps the blood through the pulmonary valve into the lungs. The blood is oxygenated in the lungs and is returned to the left atrium. The blood leaves the left atrium through the mitral valve and enters the left ventricle. The left ventricle pumps the oxygenated blood through the aortic valve to the rest of the body; it then returns to the heart via the right atrium.

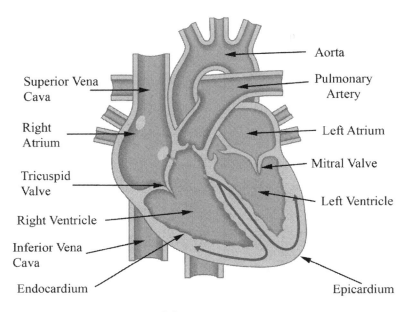

Figure 1. Basic Anatomy of the Heart

If the coronary arteries of the heart represent the "plumbing," then the conduction system of the heart represents the "wiring." Figure 2 represents the conduction system of the heart. Normal heart rate is sixty to one hundred beats per minute (bpm). *Bradycardia* is an abnormally slow heart rate, less than 60 bpm, and *tachycardia* refers to an abnormally fast heart rate, greater than 100 bpm. The sinoatrial (SA) node serves as the internal clock—or natural pacemaker—of the heart and signals the appropriate heart rate for a given situation.

Electrical-conduction system of the heart. The heart's natural pacemaker (the SA node) is located in the top-right chamber of the heart: the right atrium. The SA node sends a signal to the upper chambers (the right and left atria) and the lower chambers (the right and left ventricles) via the atrioventricular (AV) node. The AV node transmits the electrical signal to the bottom chambers via the left and right bundle branches. The left bundle branch is comprised of left-posterior and left-anterior *fascicles,* another term for divisions or branches. Often, the patient has a slow heart rate because the electrical connection between the top (the signal from the SA node) and bottom (the ventricles) of the heart is diseased; the condition is called *AV block*. The most common type of defibrillator involves placing leads in the right atrium and right ventricle.

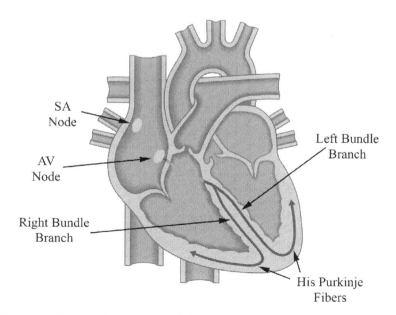

Figure 2. Conduction System of the Heart

Coronary arteries. The coronary arteries supply blood (and hence, oxygen) to the heart muscle; they course along the outside of the heart (*epicardium*). Each coronary artery supplies particular muscle territories in the heart. The left, main, coronary artery comes off the aorta and branches into the left-anterior descending (LAD) and circumflex (CX) arteries. The right coronary artery (RCA) comes off the right side of the aorta and ultimately branches into the posterolateral (PLA) and posterior descending arteries (PDA). See table 1 for blood supplies of various elements of the conduction system. One can see why an AV block is often seen during heart attacks (blockages of coronary arteries) involving the RCA, because 80 percent of patients have their AV-node blood supply provided by the RCA. In addition, a left-posterior fascicular block is uncommonly due to coronary disease because it has a dual blood supply. It would require two occluded coronary arteries (PDA and LAD septal perforators) to become blocked.

Table 1. Blood Supply to the Heart's Electrical-Conduction System

STRUCTURE	BLOOD SUPPLY (%)
SA Node	55% RCA; 35% Left Circumflex; 10% Dual
AV Node	80% RCA; 10% Left Circumflex; 10% Dual
RBB	LAD Septal Perforators, AV Nodal Branch of RCA
LBB: LAF	LAD Septal Perforators
LBB: LPF	PDA and LAD Septal Perforators

SA=sinoatrial, AV=atrioventricular, RBB=right bundle branch, LBB=left bundle branch, LAF=left-anterior fascicle, LPF=left-posterior fascicle.

Electrocardiogram (ECG or EKG). One of the most important tools that doctors have to assess the electrical function of your heart is the electrocardiogram. Figure 3 depicts a typical electrocardiogram tracing and shows how this waveform represents the electrical and pumping actions of your heart. The reason a typical ECG in your doctor's office has twelve leads (or tracings) is because this allows your doctor to better localize arrhythmias and areas of prior heart attacks as well as other structural abnormalities.

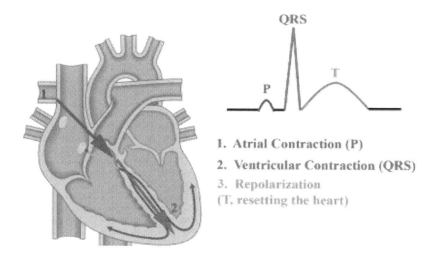

1. Atrial Contraction (P)
2. Ventricular Contraction (QRS)
3. Repolarization
(T, resetting the heart)

Figure 3. The Electrocardiogram and Its Relation to Heart Timing/ Pumping

The *P wave* corresponds to the electrical activation of the right and left atria. The right and left atria contract and pump the blood to the right and left ventricles, respectively. The *PR interval* is the time it takes for electrical activation from the SA node through the AV node to the right and left ventricles. The *QRS complex* is the electrical representation of the right and left ventricles contracting and pumping blood out of the heart. The QRS complex duration is measured to determine the type of defibrillator to be implanted (to be discussed later). The *T wave* corresponds to repolarization (or resetting of the ventricles' electrical system) prior to the next contraction of the heart. The time from the onset of the QRS complex to the end of the T wave (called the *QT interval*) can be prolonged in patients at risk for sudden cardiac death.

2
Basics of Heart Failure and Sudden Death

What is congestive heart failure? Congestive heart failure (CHF) generally means that your heart cannot pump blood as efficiently as your body needs it to. This is most commonly due to the heart's weakening and its inability to pump enough blood (called *systolic heart failure*). CHF often occurs when a patient's *ejection fraction* (EF) drops below the normal of 55 to 70 percent. In addition, a common type of heart failure (called *diastolic heart failure*) results from an inability of the heart to relax properly. Diastolic heart failure is common in elderly patients with high blood pressure. Symptoms of heart failure include:

- Shortness of breath during exertion or while lying down
- Chest pain

- Swelling (*edema*) in feet, ankles, or legs
- Irregular or fast heart rate
- Weakness and fatigue
- Reduced ability to walk or exercise
- Coughing (sometimes with pink sputum) or wheezing
- Sudden weight gain
- Loss of appetite or stomach discomfort

The appearance of these symptoms should be relayed to your doctor.

What causes heart failure? The American College of Cardiology has developed extensive guidelines for the diagnosis and treatment of heart failure (Hunt et al. 2001). A doctor who suspects heart failure may check your electrocardiogram, blood laboratories (discussed in chapter 5), and assess your ejection fraction to find the underlying cause of the heart failure. Coronary-artery blockages are the underlying cause for two-thirds of patients with heart failure (called *ischemic cardiomyopathy*). The remaining patients have heart failure caused by hypertension, heart-valve disease, heart-muscle (myocardial) disease, or toxins such as alcohol or some types of cancer medications. Sometimes patients have no obvious cause for their heart failure (called *idiopathic cardiomyopathy*).

A patient can be considered a candidate for a defibrillator several weeks to months after reversible causes of heart failure are treated, appropriate medical management has been attempted, and the patient's ejection fraction (see below) *is below 35 percent.*

Know your ejection fraction! The best single predictor for risk of sudden death (and the need for a defibrillator) is your *ejection fraction*. Ejection fraction refers to how much blood your heart pumps on every beat. The ejection fraction is most commonly measured during echocardiography (an ultrasound of your heart) or stress testing. Your ejection fraction may also be measured during a CT scan or MRI of your heart. In addition, the multigated acquisition (MUGA) scan is a special test that can be used to measure your heart's ejection fraction. Talk to your care provider about the type of test used to measure your ejection fraction. The healthy heart ejects 55 to 70 percent of the blood it can hold during every beat. Once a patient's heart pumps less than 35 percent during a typical heartbeat, the patient is considered at risk for sudden death and a candidate for a defibrillator. It must be emphasized, however, that there are several situations in which a defibrillator is recommended if the ejection fraction is greater than 35 percent; these include hypertrophic cardiomyopathy, long-QT syndrome, and other situations to be discussed in chapter 3.

What is ventricular fibrillation or ventricular tachycardia? Ventricular tachycardia refers to a very fast beating of the bottom chambers of the heart (the ventricles) and can cause low blood pressure, loss of consciousness, and even death if not treated. Ventricular fibrillation refers to an even faster beating of the bottom chambers of the heart (ventricles) and is often fatal. During a *sudden cardiac death*, when the heart goes into ventricular fibrillation, the bottom chambers just quiver and no blood is pumped. This leads to a loss of blood pressure then the loss of consciousness (called *syncope* or fainting) and then, if not stopped quickly, death. It may seem confusing, but it is possible to survive a sudden cardiac death. A person can faint because of a sudden cardiac death (e.g., ventricular fibrillation as shown in the following figure) and be revived quickly, depending on the underlying medical condition and availability of emergency personnel.

Figure 4 shows the electrocardiogram of a patient who had an episode of ventricular fibrillation while hospitalized. This patient quickly underwent an electrical *cardioversion* and had a defibrillator placed to stop further episodes of ventricular fibrillation. A cardioversion is a procedure using electricity (as in this case) or medicines to convert an abnormally fast heart rhythm to a normal rhythm.

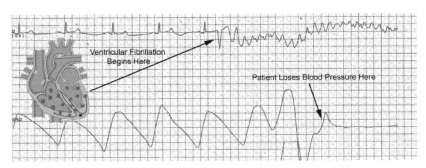

Figure 4. Ventricular Fibrillation Causing Cardiac Arrest

Is there a difference between atrial fibrillation and ventricular fibrillation? Atrial fibrillation and ventricular fibrillation are *very* different. Atrial fibrillation is the most common clinical arrhythmia encountered in cardiac electrophysiology, and it is a problem of the top chambers in your heart—that is, the atria. Approximately 5 percent of the population over sixty years old have it! If you have atrial fibrillation, your most significant risk is stroke, and the first step in treatment is deciding what type of anticoagulation is appropriate for your situation. Aspirin alone may be adequate, but you may require warfarin or one of the newer oral anticoagulants that can be used in place of warfarin (Coumadin®). The next issue is to determine how to manage the heart-rhythm abnormality itself. A *rhythm-control* strategy is in place when you are given *antiarrhythmics* (medications that help maintain a normal rhythm) to prevent atrial fibrillation from happening; this strategy is ideal for patients with severe symptoms. Antiarrhythmics include flecainide, propafenone, amiodarone, sotalol, dofetilide, and dronedarone. A *rate-control* strategy allows the presence of atrial fibrillation but prevents fast heart rates with medications to slow your heart rate; this is a good option for patients who do not feel their atrial fibrillation (three out of ten patients with atrial fibrillation may not have symptoms). Medications to help slow your heart while you are in atrial fibrillation include beta-blockers (e.g., metoprolol, atenolol, and carvedilol), calcium-channel blockers (e.g., diltiazem and verapamil), and digoxin.

The most important thing to realize is that atrial fibrillation will not be completely treated (or understood) in a single visit. Be patient with your care provider. A medicine that works for one patient may not work for another. Remember: atrial fibrillation is very different from ventricular fibrillation!

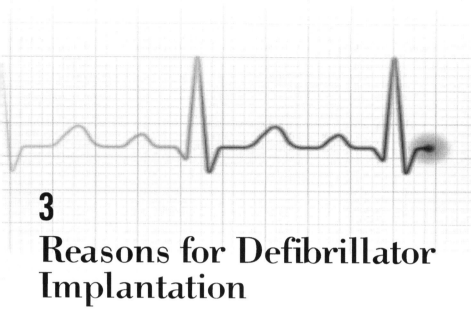

3
Reasons for Defibrillator Implantation

Introduction. Your care providers have extensive training assessing the reasons—also called *indications*—that a patient may need a defibrillator. In particular, it is very important that the benefits of defibrillator implantation outweigh the risks of the defibrillator-implant surgery (to be discussed later). The American College of Cardiology (ACC) is one of the major professional societies that develop guidelines to help care providers make educated clinical decisions based upon prior clinical studies. This is the foundation of "evidence-based" medicine: the process by which clinical ideas are tested, reported, and reevaluated to decide the most appropriate care for a particular condition.

The ACC has developed guidelines that help care providers decide when a patient would be best served by a defibrillator (Writing Committee 2008). The easiest rule to remember is this: *defibrillators are most appropriate to prevent the recurrence of a life-threatening ventricular arrhythmia (secondary prevention) or to avoid the initial occurrence of a life-threatening ventricular arrhythmia (primary prevention).*

The decision to implant a defibrillator requires evaluation of the duration of heart failure and whether or not the patient has been adequately treated for it; for example, has the patient been placed on the appropriate medications, and have coronary-artery blockages and other reversible causes of heart failure been addressed? Also, there are some diseases that may warrant defibrillator implantation even without the presence of heart failure (for example, hypertrophic cardiomyopathy, long-QT syndrome, or arrhythmogenic right-ventricular dysplasia). Some patients with psychiatric disorders may not be candidates for defibrillators because they cannot adequately follow up on device care or their conditions may be worsened by device implantations. Finally, defibrillators are not appropriate for patients who have a life expectancy of less than one year.

Survival benefits of defibrillators. Defibrillators have been shown to improve life expectancy by lowering death rates in appropriately selected patients. There have been many trials examining outcomes of patients with or without a defibrillator. Figure 5 shows a simplified version of results of defibrillator trials for both primary and secondary prevention of sudden death (a.k.a. ventricular tachycardia or fibrillation; Ezekowitz, Armstrong, and McAlister 2003).

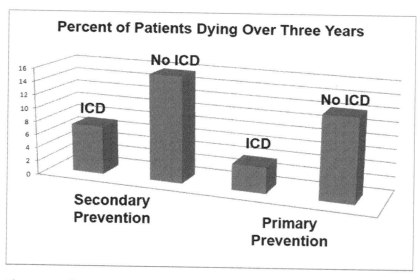

Figure 5. Effect of Defibrillators on Patient Survival

One can see lower death rates in patients who undergo defibrillator implantation for appropriate reasons. Obviously, the risks and benefits of a defibrillator implantation will depend on both the underlying medical condition and the reason (or indication) for defibrillator implantation; these issues should be discussed with your care provider.

Disease states at risk for sudden cardiac death
(Writing Committee 2008).

Coronary-artery disease. Many patients who have survived a sudden cardiac death have this disease, characterized by underlying blockages in their coronary arteries. Sometimes the first presentation of coronary-artery disease is a heart attack (sudden coronary-artery blockage) that causes cardiac arrest from ventricular fibrillation. In this setting, opening the blocked coronary artery will effectively treat the condition without a defibrillator implantation. A patient who experiences cardiac arrest or sudden death within forty-eight hours of a heart attack may not require defibrillator therapy.

Many patients have long-standing coronary-artery blockages that ultimately lead to heart failure and a reduced EF—this is called *chronic ischemic heart disease.* Another name for this reduction in EF from coronary-artery disease is *ischemic cardiomyopathy* (also see chapter 2). When a patient's EF drops below 35 percent, a defibrillator is often recommended to prevent sudden cardiac death from ventricular tachycardia or ventricular fibrillation. There are some situations where a patient with coronary disease may need to undergo a defibrillator implantation even with an EF greater than 35 percent. These situations include fainting from ventricular tachycardia or ventricular fibrillation or an electrophysiology study where a fatal arrhythmia is induced. Here is a common clinical scenario:

Common Clinical Scenario #1

A fifty-five-year-old man has had multiple heart attacks over several years and has had progressive shortness of breath despite optimal medical management. He has undergone coronary-artery-bypass surgery, and a recent catheterization reveals that while his native coronary arteries are still severely diseased, his bypass grafts are all still working properly. His EF is found to be 25 percent. Consultation with a special cardiologist (called an *electrophysiologist*) reveals that his shortness of breath is from heart failure, and it is recommended that he undergo a defibrillator implantation.

Nonischemic cardiomyopathy. Some patients get heart failure and an EF reduced to below 35 percent without any underlying coronary-artery blockages. Once all reversible causes of the patient's heart failure are ruled out, medications are used to treat the heart failure. If medications (usually given for at least three months) fail to normalize the EF and the patient still has heart-failure symptoms, a defibrillator should be considered. A defibrillator is especially important therapy in a patient with a nonischemic cardiomyopathy and an EF less than 35 percent with a history of unexplained syncope (fainting) or in a patient with documented episodes of ventricular tachycardia or ventricular fibrillation. Here is a second common clinical scenario:

Common Clinical Scenario #2

A forty-two-year-old female is diagnosed with heart failure and a depressed EF of 15 to 20 percent. She undergoes evaluation and is not found to have any other cause for heart disease (such a valve or coronary disease). Despite several months of medication, she continues to experience shortness of breath with minimal activity, her EF is still 15 to 20 percent, and her electrocardiogram reveals a left-bundle-branch block. She undergoes a biventricular defibrillator implantation, and six months later her EF improves to 50 percent.

Hypertrophic cardiomyopathy. This is a genetically inherited, heart-muscle disease that causes the heart walls to become abnormally thickened (hypertrophy). It is relatively rare (affecting only one in five hundred people), but it is the most common cause of sudden cardiac death in young patients (Writing Committee 2008). Hypertrophic cardiomyopathy should be suspected in a young patient who passes out during exercise or vigorous activity. An echocardiogram and electrocardiogram are usually performed to diagnose hypertrophic cardiomyopathy. Genetic testing may be undertaken to see if children or relatives of the patient may be at risk for this disorder. A defibrillator is especially important therapy in a patient with hypertrophic cardiomyopathy and a history of unexplained syncope (fainting) or documented episodes of ventricular tachycardia or ventricular fibrillation.

Arrhythmogenic right-ventricular dysplasia. This is another genetically inherited condition causing abnormal fat and fibrous deposits in the pumping walls of your right and sometimes left ventricles. It can cause ventricular tachycardia and ventricular fibrillation. Several factors may place patients at particularly high risk of sudden death; they include inducible ventricular tachycardia/fibrillation during an EP study, extensive or severe right-ventricular structural disease, male gender, or unexplained fainting (syncope). These patients generally benefit from defibrillator implantation.

Genetic arrhythmia syndromes. Long-QT syndrome is a genetic arrhythmia syndrome that places patients at an increased risk of sudden death. It is diagnosed by an abnormal EP study or electrocardiogram (see figure 3) that has a prolonged QT interval. There is no structural abnormality associated with this disorder; rather, the electrical system of the heart is abnormal. Treatment with medications such as beta-blockers can be effective, but patients experiencing unexplained syncope, ventricular arrhythmias, or who survive a sudden death may benefit from a defibrillator. There are other arrhythmia syndromes that may benefit from defibrillators such as idiopathic ventricular fibrillation, short-QT syndrome, Brugada syndrome, and catecholaminergic polymorphic ventricular tachycardia. Genetic testing may be undertaken to see if children or relatives of the patient may be at risk for these disorders. Consider the following, third, common clinical scenario.

Common Clinical Scenario #3

A thirty-seven-year-old female with long-QT syndrome presents to a cardiac electrophysiologist for a second opinion. She has carried a diagnosis of long-QT syndrome for over ten years and intermittently experiences palpitations and the feeling that she is going to pass out. She has been on a beta-blocker since she was told she had long-QT syndrome. A first-degree relative survived a (documented) sudden death and has a defibrillator. The patient's electrocardiogram in the office was normal, but a subsequent EP study revealed marked QT prolongation when special medications were given during the EP study. She undergoes defibrillator implantation, and subsequent genetic testing confirms long-QT syndrome.

Syncope (fainting) with ventricular tachycardia/fibrillation on electrophysiology study. If you have heart disease and have an episode of syncope, your care provider may recommend an electrophysiology study. The EP study is a procedure performed by cardiologists that specialize in heart-rhythm disorders (called *cardiac electrophysiologists*). Several catheters are placed in the femoral veins that are located in the creases of your groin. These catheters are then advanced up the veins that flow back to your heart. The catheters are then positioned using special x-rays (the process is called *fluoroscopy*) to make electrical measurements in your atrium and ventricles. In addition to these measurements, the electrophysiologist causes your heart to beat faster than normal by pacing the chambers at fast rates. If you are at risk for ventricular tachycardia or ventricular fibrillation, it is discovered during these pacing maneuvers. The arrhythmias that occur during EP studies are usually quickly terminated and may indicate the need for a defibrillator, as in the following, fourth, common clinical scenario.

Common Clinical Scenario #4

A sixty-five-year-old female is referred to her cardiologist after experiencing her first episode of fainting. Her abrupt loss of consciousness had caused her to wreck her car. She has a long history of coronary-artery disease and mitral-valve disease, but both have been surgically corrected. A defibrillator has never been recommended because her EF has always been 40 percent, and she's not had any other symptoms such as shortness of breath or palpitations (a feeling of heart racing). The cardiologist recommends an EP study to evaluate if perhaps this episode of syncope could have been an aborted sudden death. The EP study

> is positive for inducible ventricular fibrillation,
> and she undergoes a defibrillator implantation.

Miscellaneous reasons for defibrillator implantation.
The most common reasons for defibrillator implantation
were discussed in the preceding paragraphs, but there
are other situations in which defibrillators may be necessary (Writing Committee 2008).

Tachycardia-induced cardiomyopathy refers to heart failure that is caused by abnormally fast heart rhythms. Often,
supraventricular (coming from the top chambers, the atria)
tachycardias can cause heart failure. Atrial fibrillation is a
common type of a supraventricular tachycardia that can
lead to heart failure if untreated. Generally, atrial fibrillation
can be treated with medications or an EP study that uses
ablation. Ablation involves using special catheters to deliver
precise burns inside your heart to stop the arrhythmia.
Ventricular arrhythmias can also cause heart failure. Any
of these situations could lead to the need for a defibrillator.

Valvular cardiomyopathy refers to heart failure caused by
valve disease. This can be caused by disease of the aortic, mitral, tricuspid, or pulmonary valves. Stenosis refers
to a process in which blood is prevented from flowing
through the valve. Regurgitation refers to a process in
which the valve becomes damaged and fails to close
properly, and blood leaks backward through the valve.

Both valve regurgitation and stenosis can cause heart failure. If medicines or surgery cannot correct the valve disease and heart failure is irreversible, a defibrillator may be necessary.

Mixed cardiomyopathy simply refers to heart failure that is caused by a combination of any of the disease processes we have discussed.

Heart-transplant patients may be at risk of sudden death and may benefit from defibrillators.

Children, adolescents, or adults with congenital heart disease (i.e., heart defects they were born with) may require defibrillators.

Before you get a defibrillator implantation. It is important to reiterate that attempts should be made to treat your particular medical condition (if treatable) prior to considering a defibrillator. It is generally recommended that patients found to have low ejection fractions receive medication for at least three months. Three months of medications such as beta-blockers, ACE inhibitors, or angiotensin-receptor blockers are often enough to see some recovery in your ejection fraction. Other causes of reduced ejection fraction can be treated with coronary-artery stents, coronary-artery-bypass surgery, or heart-valve surgery. *It is important to talk to your care provider if your condition is reversible in any way prior to undergoing a defibrillator implantation.*

Summary. The most common indications for permanent defibrillator implantation have been discussed, including typical case scenarios. Obviously, not all patients will be textbook cases, and their symptoms may be atypical and/or overlap several categories. Therefore, it is critical for patients to engage in open dialogue with their care providers.

Other conditions that may warrant defibrillator implantation are beyond the scope of this book. Patients should get a second opinion if they are uncomfortable with their respective treatment plans or they have been diagnosed with rare disorders.

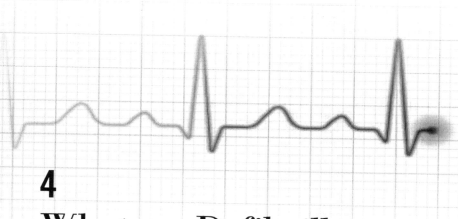

4
What are Defibrillators and How Do They Work?

Location of a transvenous defibrillator implantation. The most common implant location is underneath the left collarbone (called the *clavicle*). There are two reasons for this: 1) the majority of patients are right-handed; placing the device on the left minimizes the risk of damaging a typical patient's dominant arm; and 2) a defibrillator implantation is technically less demanding when placed on the left side. Defibrillator leads are placed into the veins of the arm that lead back to your heart. The two major veins in your arm are the cephalic and the basilica veins. These join to form the axillary vein, which then forms the subclavian vein (shown in figure 6A). This venous structure is found in both arms, though sometimes people have anatomic variants. Please note that figure 6A depicts a defibrillator but is an accurate representation of the anatomic and lead positions for a traditional pacemaker. A defibrillator is larger than a pacemaker, and the leads can be larger than traditional pacemaker leads. Remember, most defibrillators are pacemakers, but pacemakers are *not* defibrillators.

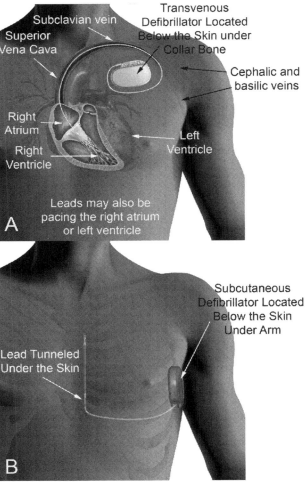

Figures 6A and 6B. Configuration of Implantable Device and Lead Implants. Image **A** depicts a defibrillator implanted via the subclavian vein. In this situation, the right-ventricular lead traverses the subclavian vein through the superior vena cava and into the right ventricle. Your doctor may choose to also place leads in the right atrium and left ventricle. Image **B** depicts a special type of defibrillator that is placed subcutaneously (under the skin) with no leads placed in the vascular system or heart. This subcutaneous defibrillator cannot perform routine pacing functions. (© 2014 Boston Scientific Corporation or its affiliates. All rights reserved. Used with permission of Boston Scientific Corporation.)

The incision is about five to eight centimeters (two to three inches) long, and the device pocket is made under the skin but above the chest muscle. The leads are placed into the subclavian vein and, ultimately, into the heart. Once the leads are placed into the heart, they are then sewn into place in the device pocket and connected to the defibrillator. The defibrillator is placed into the device pocket—with the remaining portion of the leads coiled under the defibrillator—and the pocket is then sewn shut.

Location of a subcutaneous defibrillator implantation. A relatively new defibrillator does not involve leads placed through the chest wall into the venous system (see Figure 6B). It is called *subcutaneous* because the device and lead are placed under the skin of the chest wall. It can be used to shock a patient out of ventricular tachycardia or ventricular fibrillation but does not offer the ability to provide routine pacing of the atrium or ventricle. It may offer fewer complications because there are no leads placed into the venous system or attached to the heart. Your doctor will have more information if this is an appropriate option for you. Most of the discussion in this book will pertain to transvenous defibrillator systems.

What are the elements of a defibrillator? The defibrillator itself is comprised of a battery, circuitry that serves as the brain, and a header that connects the leads to the defibrillator itself. Figures 7A, 7B, and 7C show typical sizes of defibrillators (7A), basic lead types (7B), and the internal construction of a defibrillator (7C).

A common clinical question:

Is there a difference between pacemakers and defibrillators?

Almost all defibrillators are pacemakers, but pacemakers are *not* defibrillators. Defibrillators can also involve placing leads into the right atrium and ventricles. These leads can also be used to prevent the heart from beating too slowly (i.e., they can function as a pacemaker), but they have an additional role. The defibrillator lead in the right ventricle allows the device to sense a possibly fatal arrhythmia. If a fatal arrhythmia is detected by the device, it can shock the patient back to life! This is very similar to what you see on TV, except that there are no paddles applied to the chest wall; the device leads permit us to deliver over seven hundred volts directly to the

---

inside of a patient's heart. Again, most defibrillators are pacemakers, but pacemakers are *not* defibrillators. As an illustration, there is a new defibrillator that is placed under the skin of the chest (i.e., *subcutaneously*) with no leads placed into the heart. This subcutaneous defibrillator cannot perform routine pacing.

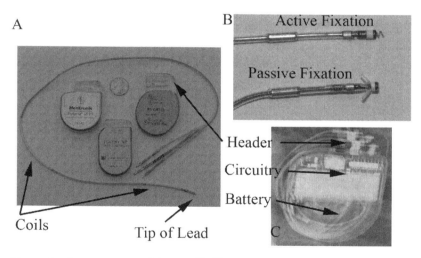

Figure 7. Components of the Defibrillator (Sizes of Typical Defibrillators [A], Lead Types [B], and Defibrillator Construction [C]) The different sizes of defibrillators are shown compared to the size of a quarter. A sample defibrillator lead is also shown (7A). Active- and passive-fixation leads are shown (7B). An x-ray showing the cross section of a defibrillator with battery, circuitry, and header to attach leads (7C).

The size of the defibrillator is based mostly on the size of the battery and header. The headers can vary in size depending upon the number of leads attached to the defibrillator; a defibrillator with a single lead generally has a smaller footprint than a defibrillator with three leads attached. The defibrillator leads have special "coils" built into the lead; these coils are used by the defibrillator to shock the heart if necessary. Think of these coils as smaller, inside-the-body versions of the paddles you see emergency personnel hold against a person's chest when using an external defibrillator. The two types of leads are called *active* and *passive fixation*. Fixation describes how the tip of the defibrillator lead is attached to the heart. Figure 7B shows active-fixation (screw) and passive-fixation lead (silicone tines). The active-fixation lead is comprised of a tiny screw that is rotated to engage the inner wall of the heart (endocardium). This is the most common type of lead implanted in the right atrium and ventricle. The passive-fixation lead has soft plastic barbs/tines at the tip; these tines anchor the tip of the lead to the heart. There are many intricate "nooks and crannies" (called _trabeculations_) that line the inside of your heart. These trabeculations allow passive-fixation leads to anchor in place. These leads are not as common, because they can be technically challenging to implant. There is some evidence that these passive-fixation leads are safer in extremely elderly patients, because they are less likely to cause a perforation (hole in the heart). All current left-ventricular leads used in heart-failure pacemakers (resynchronization devices) are passive—except for one model (Starfix™, Medtronic, Inc., Minneapolis, MN) that has a mechanism to prevent dislodgement. Finally, a defibrillator RV lead is shown, and it includes two coils; the defibrillator delivers the shock through these coils.

Defibrillator to help treat heart-failure patients. Patients receiving defibrillators are obviously at risk of sudden death and often have severe heart failure. They can have dyssynchronous contraction (the right and left ventricles do not pump at the same time) that causes heart-failure symptoms such as shortness of breath and leg swelling. This may require an additional lead to be placed into the coronary sinus that can pace the left side of the heart (the left ventricle). This lead in the left ventricle is used to resynchronize the pumping action of the heart so that the right and left ventricles pump at the same time. The coronary sinus is paper thin and very easily perforated, and requires great care and caution to implant. Indeed, left-ventricular leads can be technically demanding to implant, and they may add hours to a defibrillator implant. Figure 6A also shows the approximate position of a lead (LV lead at tip of arrow) that is used to pace the lower-left chamber of the heart (called the *left ventricle*).

How are defibrillators programmed? Your care providers communicate with your defibrillator to give and get information either via a wand placed over the device or wirelessly (now available on most devices). A *programmer* is used to check the device to make sure the leads are functioning properly and to program pacing and therapy features on the defibrillator. This is called *interrogation*. Defibrillators are programmed to pace, depending on the condition the doctors are trying to treat. Table 2 describes the different modes that your defibrillator may be programmed to. Defibrillators can be programmed to pace at different rates determined by your doctor. There is also a way to program your defibrillator to pace at a rate that matches your activity level. This is called *rate-responsive* programming.

Table 2. Different Types of Defibrillators

TYPE OF DEFIBRILLATOR	LEADS REQUIRED	HOW DOES IT WORK?	CLINICAL SCENARIO
Single-chamber	Right-ventricle lead	A single right-ventricular lead is placed into the heart. The device can pace the bottom chamber if needed as well as deliver shocks.	These devices are implanted in patients who do not need sophisticated pacing features.
Dual-chamber (Ventricular)	Right-atrial and right-ventricular leads.	Both right-atrial and right-ventricular pacing is possible with this device.	A patient who has risks for sudden death but also has heart block and needs atrial and ventricular pacing features.
Biventricular	Right-atrial, right-ventricular, and left-ventricular leads.	Leads are placed into the right ventricle, right atrium, and into the left ventricle via the coronary sinus.	These heart-failure patients are not only at risk of sudden death but also need a special type of pacing called *resynchronization*.

Subcutaneous-only System	Lead tunneled under the skin of the chest. The device itself is placed under the skin of the lateral chest under the arm.	A single lead is placed under the skin of the chest wall. The device can deliver shocks to terminate arrhythmias but cannot provide routine pacing.	Patients at risk for sudden death who do not need (or cannot get) implantable, transvenous leads or do not need routine pacing.

The most important feature of defibrillator programming is to deliver therapies to terminate a life-threatening arrhythmia such as ventricular tachycardia or ventricular fibrillation. Essentially, the defibrillator has very sophisticated software algorithms to detect abnormal heart rhythms and decide if they are potentially life-threatening. This is done primarily by selecting a heart rate (such as two hundred beats per minute) that is above the normal fast heart rate that may be found during periods of heavy exertion. The device then analyzes several other features of the heart rhythm: is it regular or irregular, was it a gradual or abrupt onset, and are the atria and ventricles beating at the same rate? These features allow the device to make the most accurate assessment of the abnormal heart rhythm. If the device decides that the arrhythmia is life-threatening, it may attempt to stop (or *terminate*) the arrhythmia. Often the device will deliver a very powerful shock to terminate the arrhythmia. Most patients are unconscious when this happens, but, if they are awake, the shock can be felt and may be quite painful. See chapters 9 and 10 for more discussions about defibrillator shocks.

Some patients have life-threatening arrhythmias that can be painlessly stopped. Antitachycardia pacing refers to a special type of pacing that the patient cannot feel, but it can stop the arrhythmia. I often program the defibrillator to perform antitachycardia pacing in an attempt to painlessly terminate an arrhythmia prior to delivering a potentially painful (albeit lifesaving) defibrillator shock. Every patient is different, and it is very important to talk to your physician about the type of device and type of programming that are best for your particular situation.

What is a wearable defibrillator? Sometimes your doctor will worry that you are at risk for sudden death, but you don't meet the necessary medical reasons for an implantable defibrillator. A wearable defibrillator can be used until a final decision is made regarding an implantable defibrillator. A patient with newly diagnosed heart failure that has not yet been treated with medications may have to wait for three months to see if the heart recovers with medications. Another common situation is a patient who had a heart attack that was successfully treated with a stent or even coronary-artery-bypass surgery; it can take weeks to months for the heart to recover. Finally, if device implantation has to be delayed because of infection, the wearable defibrillator can be used until the infection has cleared.

While you are waiting for heart function to possibly recover or an infection to resolve, your doctor may offer you a wearable external defibrillator (LifeVest™, Zoll Medical Corporation, Pittsburgh, PA) to help protect you from sudden cardiac death. The wearable defibrillator is a specially equipped vest that can detect and terminate ventricular arrhythmias. You wear it all the time except while showering. Its cost is usually covered by insurance if your condition merits its use. Ask your doctor if you are a candidate for this type of device.

How does a defibrillator stop a life-threatening arrhythmia? Figure 8 shows a typical episode in a patient with a defibrillator. The patient developed ventricular tachycardia (VT), and the defibrillator's software was programmed to recognize it. In this case, the defibrillator was able to rapidly pace the ventricles and stop (terminate) the VT. This rapid pacing is called *antitachycardia pacing* (ATP) and the patient generally does not feel it. If the initial ATP is unsuccessful, the defibrillator may try faster ATP or will resort to a shock.

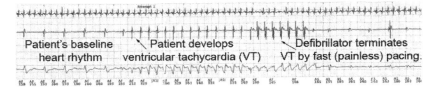

Figure 8. Defibrillator Stopping a Lethal Arrhythmia (ventricular tachycardia, VT). This figure shows a recording from a patient's defibrillator. The first part of the recording shows the patient's baseline heart rhythm (this patient happens to be in permanent atrial fibrillation). The patient then develops VT, which, if left untreated, could lead to death. The defibrillator recognizes the VT and then paces the ventricle very fast, which painlessly terminates the VT. A shock from the defibrillator may not be painless if the patient is awake.

Are defibrillator shocks painful? Believe it or not, some patients may not pass out (or lose consciousness) during an arrhythmia. So if the patient is awake during an episode of VT/VF, then, yes, the shock may be painful. I often describe this shock to a patient as feeling "like a horse kicked you in the chest." It must be noted, though, that often patients do pass out during an arrhythmia and are unconscious when the defibrillator delivers the therapies (either ATP or a shock). See chapters 9 and 10 to learn what to do if your defibrillator delivers a shock.

When should I have the pacing features of my defibrillator turned on? As we've discussed, most defibrillators are pacemakers, but pacemakers are not defibrillators. Defibrillators implanted solely to protect a patient from sudden death will usually be programmed to pace only if heart rate drops below forty (usually) beats per minute. Many patients undergoing defibrillator implantation have electrical-conduction-system disease, which may require their doctors to program their defibrillators to function as pacemakers.

Following are some common reasons your doctor may choose to activate the pacing features of your defibrillator.

Sinoatrial node dysfunction. The sinus node is the heart's pacemaker—or metronome. As you age, the pacemaker may beat too fast, which can be treated with medicines that slow the heart rate. These medicines include beta-blockers, such as: metoprolol, atenolol, propranolol, or carvedilol. More often, however, sinus-node dysfunction can cause your heart to beat too slowly. You can be symptomatic because the heart is beating too slowly (symptomatic bradycardia) or does not beat fast enough during exercise (chronotropic incompetence). In situations where the heart does not beat fast enough or where medications to treat fast heart rates cause the heart to beat too slowly, pacing can be used to reestablish a normal heart rate.

In my practice, I find a surprising number of patients who have been experiencing symptomatic chronotropic incompetence. As a person exercises, he or she is more and more dependent upon heart rate to increase the amount of blood that is pumped by the heart (cardiac output). A rule of thumb is that a person's maximum heart rate is 220 minus the person's age. There are several ways to assess chronotropic incompetence: 1) inability to achieve maximum heart rate, 2) delay in reaching maximum heart rate, 3) inadequate submaximal heart rate or recovery heart rate, and 4) excessive variation in heart rate during exercise (rate instability; Lukl et al. 1999). Chronotropic incompetence has been found in 11 to 26 percent of patients undergoing stress tests, and it is associated with an increased risk of death—likely associated with underlying coronary-artery disease (Lauer et al. 1999).

Acquired atrioventricular block in adults. The most important thing to remember is that pacing is most beneficial when you have symptoms attributable to conduction delay through the AV node. Atrioventricular block refers to conduction delay between the top (atria) and bottom (ventricles) chambers of the heart. There are several different types of AV block, and these include: first-degree AV block, second-degree AV block, and complete heart block. First-degree heart block represents a simple delay in the AV node; it is generally harmless and does not require pacing. Second-degree heart block occurs when electrical impulses are intermittently blocked between the atria and ventricles. It can be a normal, nonfatal finding in patients (e.g., Type I second-degree AV block) but can also cause symptoms and may require pacing (e.g., Type II second-degree AV block). Third-degree AV block (also called *complete heart block*) occurs when the electrical connection between the atria and ventricles is disrupted, and the chambers beat independently with no electrical connection. *Most often, third-degree heart block requires permanent pacing.*

Chronic bifascicular block. Bifascicular block refers to block below the AV node in the right and left bundle branches. The left bundle branch is comprised of the left-posterior and left-anterior fascicles. You can have alternating right- and left-bundle-branch blocks and be at risk of complete heart block; pacing is generally recommended. If you have bifascicular block and show evidence of complete heart block or second-degree (type 2) AV block, you will likely benefit from pacing support.

Hypersensitive carotid-sinus syndrome. Hypersensitive carotid-sinus syndrome is also known as carotid-sinus hypersensitivity (CSH). CSH is an extreme reflex response to carotid-sinus stimulation: rubbing the carotid artery where it runs next to the Adam's apple. There are two components of the reflex (Writing Committee 2008):

1) cardioinhibitory response, resulting from increased parasympathetic-nervous-system tone, is manifested by a slowing of the sinus rate or prolongation of the PR interval and advanced AV block—alone or in combination; and (2) vasodepressor response, which stems from a reduction in sympathetic-nervous-system activity that results in loss of vascular tone and hypotension (drop in blood pressure) independent of heart rate.

It is very important for your doctor to determine if you have cardioinhibitory response to carotid-sinus stimulation when deciding if pacing is warranted. A pause of more than three seconds—causing low blood pressure or fainting—is suggestive of CSH. Pacing support in patients with excessive cardioinhibitory response to carotid-sinus massage is usually effective at relieving symptoms. Carotid-sinus hypersensitivity in elderly patients is also associated with carotid vascular disease (O'Mahony 1995), and it may be associated with 45 to 50 percent of elderly patients who present with falls (O'Mahony 1995; Crilley et al. 1997).

Miscellaneous reasons for pacing support of defibrillator patients. The most common reasons for pacing support were discussed in the preceding paragraphs, but there are other situations in which pacing support may be necessary in defibrillator patients (Writing Committee 2008).

Patients who have had heart transplants may have slow heart rates (bradycardia) that respond to pacing.

Neuromuscular diseases—such as muscular and myotonic dystrophies—may cause progressive conduction-system disease, leading to complete heart block. *Patients with sleep apnea* (breathing stops during sleep) may have slow heart rates (sinus bradycardia) or even long pauses while sleeping.

Sarcoidosis causes granulomas (abnormal collections of immune cells) to form that have heart involvement in 25 percent of patients, and heart block may develop in 30 percent of these patients. Depending upon the clinical situation, patients with sarcoidosis may benefit from pacing support.

Pacing can be used for the prevention and termination of heart-rhythm abnormalities. A variety of atrial and ventricular arrhythmias can be prevented and terminated by pacing. In particular, patients with long-QT syndrome may benefit from pacing, because many rhythm disturbances are initiated by slow heart rates.

Atrial fibrillation is a common rhythm disturbance that may require pacing support. The vast majority of atrial-fibrillation patients require medicines to slow down their hearts during periods of atrial fibrillation. There are patients who have atrial fibrillation with very slow heart rates, or who are taking medications to control fast heart rates (tachycardia) during atrial fibrillation and experience very slow heart rates (bradycardia) when normal rhythm returns. This is called *tachycardia-bradycardia syndrome.* These patients with atrial fibrillation may benefit from pacing.

It is important to remember that the very patients at risk for sudden death because of underlying heart disease are at risk for conduction-system disease and the need for pacing support. It is important to talk to one's doctor before a defibrillator implantation and ask what (if any) pacing support will be programmed into the defibrillator.

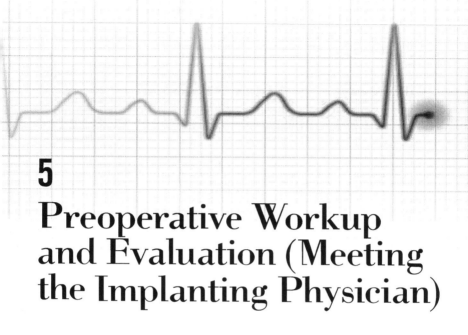

5
Preoperative Workup and Evaluation (Meeting the Implanting Physician)

Introduction. The first important element of the evaluation for a defibrillator is the type of doctor who will be performing the defibrillator implantation. All doctors have years of training built upon a foundation of patient evaluation that permits a thorough, yet concise, summary of a patient and his or her symptoms, medical history, and differential diagnosis. The differential diagnosis consists of the possible diagnoses (in order of likelihood) that can explain the patient's symptom constellation. That being said, there is a wide variety of doctors—with a wide variety of training backgrounds—who can implant defibrillators.

- A *cardiologist* is an Internal Medicine medicine doctor whose training involves four years of under-graduate college, four years of medical school, three years of Internal Medicine residency, and three years of Cardiology fellowship. Many cardiologists are board certified in Internal Medicine and Cardiology.
- An *electrophysiologist* (EP) is a subspecialized cardiologist who performs heart-rhythm evaluations and electrophysiology-device—such as pacemakers and defibrillators—implants. Typical training involves the same training as a cardiologist—plus an additional two years of Electrophysiology (Heart Rhythm) fellowship. During this electrophysiology fellowship, an EP focuses exclusively on pacemaker and defibrillator implantation as well as long-term care of these devices. In addition, an EP is trained in all aspects of heart-rhythm evaluation and care, including electrophysiology studies and heart ablations to cure various arrhythmias. Many EPs are board certified in Internal Medicine, Cardiology, and Clinical Cardiac Electrophysiology.
- *General and cardiothoracic surgeons* can sometimes implant defibrillators. Surgeons undergo five years of a general-surgery residency and heart surgeons will do an additional two to three years of heart surgery. Their training involves the implant procedure with no long-term follow-up defibrillator care (except in few instances).

Questions to Ask Your Doctor before Surgery

1. What is your training background?

There is evidence that physician training (specifically, board certification or board eligibility in clinical cardiac electrophysiology) may result in lower rates of complications such as lead dislodgement (Curtis et al. 2009; Cheng et al. 2010).

2. How many implants have you done?

Doctors who perform more defibrillator implants seem to have fewer complications than doctors who only perform a handful a year. Specifically, higher-volume (greater than twelve implants per year) versus lower-volume operators (fewer than twelve implants per year) have also demonstrated lower rates of complication (Parsonnet, Bernstein, and Lindsay 1989).

3. What have your complications been?

This question can be especially enlightening, because it will give you an idea of whether the doctor has looked at his or her outcomes. A doctor who tells you that he or she has had no complications is misinformed or has not done enough procedures. Any doctor who performs procedures has complications, and a doctor who cares about patient outcomes will have done due diligence to minimize complications from happening again. That being said, there is generally no way to have no complications, but it is important to choose a doctor who has in-depth knowledge of possible complications.

4. What type of pacemaker will be implanted, and why?

A rule of thumb is that more complex devices (dual-chamber vs. single-ventricular-chamber defibrillators) have been associated with higher rates of complications. However, there are also data that do not demonstrate increased rates of complications in dual-chamber devices (Williams and Stevenson 2012). In addition, the placement of a left-ventricular lead may entail more time and risk than other types of leads.

I have seen cardiologists, electrophysiologists, and surgeons with exceptional (and catastrophic) outcomes of defibrillator-implant surgery. There are *several questions you can ask the implanting physician* to assess his or her chances of a successful defibrillator with low risk of complications.

History of present illness (HPI). The most important element of evaluating a patient is an open discussion to determine the present illness. It is estimated that over 80 percent of patients can be diagnosed just by obtaining an accurate history from the patient (Hampton et al. 1975). One of the most important aspects in the evaluation of a patient for a defibrillator is whether or not the patient has been appropriately treated and is at risk for sudden cardiac death. Symptoms such as loss of consciousness (syncope), dizziness, shortness of breath, chest pain, palpitations, or exertional fatigue can all be related to heart-rhythm disorders requiring a defibrillator.

Typical Patient HPI: This is a seventy-two-year-old, white female who has had eleven episodes of sudden loss of consciousness over the past four years. She has had seizure activity witnessed by others, and, under the care of her primary-care physician, neurologist, and general cardiologist, she has been started on an antiseizure medicine. She continues to experience episodes of syncope. Each episode involves a short period of dizziness and blacking out. This is followed by a loss of consciousness. These episodes, more often than not, are abrupt in their onset, occur without much warning, and have resulted in injury at times. They can occur while the patient is seated or standing. They do not appear to be related to meals, dehydration, emotional stress, or any other obvious cause. There are no related symptoms such as chest pain, shortness of breath, or rapid heartbeat.

Common elements of the history of present illness (HPI). We can describe the HPI using seven categories to encompass all elements of the history. COLDER-AS is a mnemonic used to ensure that all the right questions are asked when evaluating a patient: Character, Onset, Location, Duration, Exacerbating Factors, Relieving Factors, and Associated Symptoms (see table 3).

Character concerns the subjective elements of the symptom or problem. Each of the remaining elements is then used to describe the particular issue for a complete description. The HPI can be gathered from anyone familiar with patient care. Physician extenders—such as nurse practitioners, physician assistants, nurses, or medical assistants—may gather this background information. It is not so much how the information is obtained; rather, that *all* the information is obtained.

Table 3. Major Elements in the History of Present Illness

Character	Pressure, burn, ache.
Onset	Circumstances/timing of symptoms.
Location	Where is the pain felt, and is it felt in any other locations?
Duration	How long have the symptoms been present and how long do they last?
Exacerbating factors	What has the patient done to aggravate the symptom (walking, sitting, standing, eating, drinking, etc.)?
Relieving factors	What has the patient done to relieve the symptom (deep breathing, cold water, nitroglycerin, belching, aspirin, etc.)?
Associated **S**ymptoms	What are the symptoms that the patient notices to occur at same time as the main issue? (Examples include: shortness of breath, heart racing, sweating, nausea, vomiting, etc.)

Past medical and surgical history (PMH). The past medical and surgical history helps to "risk-stratify" patients. Elements of a patient history—including prior heart attacks (myocardial infarction or MI), congestive heart failure (CHF), or arrhythmias such as ventricular tachycardia/fibrillation and atrial fibrillation—suggest underlying heart disease and possibly increased risk of sudden cardiac death. In fact, there are other, noncardiac medical problems that can hint at a possible cardiac condition that may indicate the need for a defibrillator. Peripheral vascular disease (blockages in arteries such as the carotids in the neck or arteries in the legs) can also indicate that heart disease is present. Not only can coronary arteries get plaques (or fatty blockages), but the heart's conduction and muscle system can also be diseased by a buildup of calcification and/or fibrous scar tissue.

Social history. The "social" history is used to obtain details of a person's life that are not purely medical. Personal habits such as the use of tobacco (causing vascular disease), alcohol, and illicit drugs—which are toxic to the heart muscle and cause heart-rhythm abnormalities—raise the suspicion of serious heart problems. Additionally, personal stresses—such as deaths in the family, marital issues, or the loss of a job—can increase stress. Many heart-rhythm abnormalities are exacerbated by increased stress, decreased sleep, caffeine, alcohol, or nicotine. Conversely, regular exercise, a healthy diet and sleep habits, smoking cessation, and weight loss can decrease heart-rhythm abnormalities.

Allergies. Obviously, your doctors should be aware of any drug allergy or prior, concerning reaction to any medication. Often the first exposure to a medication causes a minor reaction, but the second exposure can lead to a fatal allergic reaction (called *anaphylaxis*). It is also important to let your doctor know if you have any reactions to other substances. Knowing of a prior reaction to intravenous contrast agents (such as during a CT scan or cardiac catheterization) or latex gloves can enable your doctors to avoid using these agents or give preventive medications (called *prophylaxis*) so an adverse reaction is minimized. Prophylaxis may include the use of steroids and antihistamines. Steroids such as prednisone or hydrocortisone are often used preoperatively. In addition, antihistamines like diphenhydramine (Benadryl®) and famotidine (Pepcid®) are given to reduce the severity of a possible allergic reaction.

Family history. The saying, "an apple does not fall far from the tree," is used to emphasize the importance of family history. We are trained to specifically ask for family histories of heart disease and the ages at which it occurred. The relative must be a blood relative (not an in-law), and we are mainly concerned with *first-degree relatives,* namely, mother, father, sister, and brother. Common heart problems that can be transmitted across generations include coronary-artery disease, heart attacks, atrial fibrillation, and sudden deaths.

Sudden cardiac death refers to an unexpected (and sometimes at a very young age) death that was likely related to the heart. Additional family histories that may suggest sudden cardiac deaths include "unexplained" seizure disorders or drownings in relatives who knew how to swim. During a sudden cardiac death, the heart muscle stops pumping, causing the brain to experience a lack of oxygen and possible seizure. Family members that have sudden cardiac deaths (and miraculously recover in seconds) may be misdiagnosed with seizure disorders. In addition, some conditions that can cause sudden cardiac death are triggered by vigorous exertion (e.g., long-QT syndrome); if a person with such a condition was swimming when a sudden cardiac death occurred, the death may be mistakenly called a drowning.

Physical exam (including vital signs). Vital signs include heart rate (heartbeats per minute), blood pressure, respiratory rate (breaths per minute), and pulse oximetry (pulse ox), which measures the oxygen content of blood.

Heart rate: A normal range of resting heart rates is sixty to one hundred beats per minute (bpm). Bradycardia refers to a heart rate less than 60 bpm, but sometimes very physically fit people can have normally slow resting heart rates less than 60 bpm. Tachycardia refers to a heart rate more than 100 bpm. Generally, your heart rate accelerates to between 100 and 120 bpm during a brisk walk or step-climbing (called *sinus tachycardia*), and this is a normal response to exercise. An abnormally slow response to exercise—the inability to get heart rate above 100 bpm with associated chest pain or shortness of breath—can indicate sinus-node dysfunction and is called *chronotropic incompetence*. Abnormally fast heart rates can indicate abnormal heart rhythms that need medical treatment. The following box describes a very common arrhythmia that can result in significant heart-rate variation.

What is atrial fibrillation? Atrial fibrillation (AF) is the most common arrhythmia seen in a typical electro-physiology practice and often presents with an abnormal or irregular heart rate. Almost 5 percent (five out of one hundred) of patients aged older than sixty years have AF, and the percentage increases almost 0.5 percent per year until by eighty years of age, up to 15 percent of people may have AF.

Atrial fibrillation refers to the top chambers of the heart (the right and left atria) fibrillating (or beating rapidly) at 300–400 bpm. This rapid beating is transmitted to the lower pumping chambers of the heart (ventricles) and causes most of the symptoms attributed to AF, such as palpitations, heart racing, chest pain, or shortness of breath. The most concerning aspect of AF—aside from the afore-mentioned symptoms—is the risk of stroke (blood clots sent to the brain). Atrial fibrillation causes the atria to stop contracting and just quiver. This loss of pumping can lead to blood-clot formation in an atrium. The diagnosis of AF (or atrial flutter, a closely related heart-rhythm disorder) should lead you to a discussion with your doctor about anticoagulation to prevent the development of strokes.

Blood pressure: The goal blood pressure in most patients is 120 over 80. The top number is called the *systolic* blood pressure, and the bottom number is called the *diastolic* blood pressure. When a patient has elevated blood pressure, diet and exercise can often normalize blood pressure. Sometimes, diet and exercise are not enough, and most doctors treat blood pressures above 140 over 90 with medication. Recent research suggests that extremely elderly patients (age greater than eighty years) may have a higher target blood pressure.

Respiratory rate: The respiratory rate refers to how often a person breathes in one minute. The normal rate is approximately eight to fourteen breaths per minute. Shortness of breath (or difficulty breathing) is often associated with an increased respiratory rate.

Pulse oximetry: Pulse oximetry is used to determine the oxygen saturation in the blood. Normal oxygen saturation is greater than 95 percent. Sometimes, heart patients can have abnormal (low) pulse oximetry readings due to the presence of heart failure (or COPD).

Weight: Weight is important to obtain, because patients who have heart failure will often gain weight. Close monitoring of weight can allow a patient to alert his or her doctor of an impending heart-failure exacerbation. Generally, rapid weight gain (or loss) of more than two to three pounds in several days corresponds to fluid weight. In addition, abnormally high or low body weights may place patients at higher risk of defibrillator-implant complications.

Pertinent studies. There are many tests that the implanting physician will want to obtain prior to defibrillator implantation. A *chest radiograph,* or chest x-ray, is obtained to ensure that the lungs and heart are in suitable condition for defibrillator implantation. In addition, the baseline chest x-ray will be used as a comparison to determine if there has been any complication from the defibrillator implantation. The *electrocardiogram* (EKG) is obviously obtained to evaluate for any heart-rhythm disorders or electrical-system blockages. An echocardiogram (*echo* for short) is used to assess for any decline in heart-pumping function (ejection fraction or EF) as well as to assess for heart-chamber sizes and any valve disease. *Stress tests* may be performed prior to proceeding with defibrillator implantation. Reasons for stress tests include: 1) to see if symptoms such as chest pain or shortness of breath are due to underlying coronary-artery blockages or 2) to assess an adequate heart-rate response to exercise. If there is an inadequate heart-rate response to exercise, your doctor may place a lead in the atrium to permit the defibrillator to pace your heart during periods of activity (called *rate-response programming*, see chapter 4 to learn about defibrillator programming). Finally, *baseline blood laboratories*—such as kidney function, blood counts, and blood-coagulation studies—are performed to make sure the defibrillator implantation can be performed safely.

Preoperative risk assessment. As with all surgical procedures, recognizing and managing existing medical problems (a.k.a. comorbid conditions) preoperatively helps to mitigate the risks during and immediately after defibrillator implantation. Most patients undergoing defibrillator implantation have heart failure and other structural heart disease and cardiac conduction-system disease, which means that there is an inherently high-risk population of patients frequently served in the EP lab. Indeed, congestive heart failure (CHF) increases the risk of all surgery. A decreased ejection fraction has been found to be a predictor of perioperative complications, with the highest-risk group being those with an EF less than 35 percent: the very patients brought to the lab for defibrillators! Preprocedural management of CHF is integral to the safety of the procedure. Patients certainly should not be in a state of decompensated heart failure.

Infection (Williams and Stevenson 2012). Patients who present with systemic infection and positive blood cultures carry the highest risk of infection (Tarakji et al. 2010). Infection of implantable devices is one of the most feared complications due to the dismal prognosis of untreated infections and risk of device removal. Often, we are asked to evaluate patients who may be at risk for sudden death (especially if they have had fainting or were resuscitated after having a sudden death) when they also happen to have an infection—such as pneumonia and urinary-tract infections—as well as after heart surgery. Preimplant evaluation for potential sources of infection is critical. The estimated rate of infection of permanent defibrillator leads is between 1 and 2 percent; however, the range is from under 1 percent to greater than 10 percent. Device infection requiring removal was correlated to fever within twenty-four hours of device implant, temporary pacing prior to implant, and early reintervention for lead revision or hematoma (collection of blood under the incision) evacuation (Klug et al. 2007). The likelihood of infection (of pacemaker implants in this particular study) was nearly doubled by the patient having undergone placement of a temporary pacemaker. The association with temporary intravenous-pacing wires certainly implies an association with any indwelling lines in patients under consideration for a defibrillator—including central and peripherally inserted central catheter (PICC) lines. The duration of hospitalization prior to implant was not correlated to higher risk of infection. Infections were generally not related to new device implantation and perioperative antibiotic prophylaxis. Believe it or not, the use of perioperative antibiotics is considered controversial; however, I generally use postoperative antibiotics for five days after defibrillator implantation.

Use of contrast agents during defibrillator implantation (Williams and Stevenson 2012). Bones show up very well on x-rays, however, soft structures such as blood vessels and the heart do not. Therefore, blood vessels and heart structure are highlighted by *contrast*, a clear liquid designed for that use, during defibrillator implantation. The implanting physician will use fluoroscopy to guide the implant procedure. Fluoroscopy is a special type of imaging that allows us to perform x-rays while the patient or the heart is moving. Fluoroscopy allows us to watch catheters and leads moving in the blood vessels and the heart so that we can place them in the correct location. A typical use of contrast for a defibrillator implantation is during a subclavian venography. Subclavian venography is done to ensure that a person's subclavian vein is not blocked, so that a defibrillator can be implanted safely. If we encounter a blocked left subclavian vein on venography, we can change the implant to the right side prior to making an incision.

Contrast-induced nephropathy (CIN). Contrast-induced nephropathy (kidney failure) is a surprisingly common complication if radiocontrast is given during a procedure; CIN can occur in 15 percent of cases. It is a decline in kidney function (assessed by checking the blood level of creatinine) that typically peaks at forty-eight to seventy-two hours after exposure. Creatinine may remain above baseline for seven to fourteen days. Naturally, the best way to avoid this complication is to abstain from its use. Single-, dual-, and biventricular-lead defibrillator systems can safely be implanted without the use of contrast at all. Prior data from our Heart Rhythm Center (Williams et al. 2010) revealed that contrast was used in 101 out of 114 (88.6 percent) of the defibrillator implants. No contrast was used for generator changes, and there were no contrast reactions. Cardiac resynchronization therapy (CRT) for heart failure may require contrast agents to define the coronary-sinus

(CS) anatomy. Coronary-sinus lead placement can often be performed successfully without the use of contrast in patients at risk of contrast-induced nephropathy (Williams et al. 2010).

The vast majority of patients undergoing CRT implants are patients with heart failure and its associated comorbidities—which very frequently include diabetes and chronic kidney disease. Therefore, a working knowledge and respect for these agents is a necessity. There are several things I may do to limit the danger of kidney damage; they include 1) using a very weak, diluted contrast agent, 2) aggressively hydrating the patient (especially one with kidney disease at baseline; hydration can usually be achieved with four to six glasses of water the evening before the procedure), and 3) holding medications that can worsen kidney damage during the procedure (for example, ACE inhibitors, angiotensin-receptor blockers, and NSAIDS can be held the day prior and day of exposure, and be resumed twenty-four hours after exposure), and medications such as sodium bicarbonate and N-acetylcysteine (Mucomyst®) can be given prior to defibrillator implantation. Treatment of CIN is largely supportive (generally resolves on its own) and infrequently requires short-term dialysis.

Contrast allergies. Immediate life-threatening allergic (anaphylactic) reactions—including angioedema (face and throat swelling), bronchospasm (lung spasm), arterial hypotension (low blood pressure), and shock—can occur within minutes of and up to sixty minutes after injection of IV

contrast (Marcos and Thomsen 2001). The reported incidence of severe immediate reactions to ionic contrast material is 0.1–0.4 percent, and with the newer, nonionic, and
low-osmolar or iso-osmolar contrast, it is 0.02–0.04 percent. But death rates from the two materials do not differ
(Brockow et al. 2005). Patients with even mild anaphylac-
toid (immediate) reactions should be considered high risk in
future contrast administration.

It is common practice to premedicate with corticosteroids
with or without histamine (H1) blockers (e.g., Pepcid®) in
patients with histories of moderate or severe immediate
reactions—despite the fact that randomized trials com-
paring pretreatment strategies are severely lacking. Prior
to any procedure that may involve contrast administration, *it is essential that you inform your doctor about any
history of previous contrast reaction, asthma, renal insuffi-
ciency, diabetes, and metformin therapy* (Royal College of
Radiologists 2010). Routine premedication of all patients
who receive contrast is probably not warranted, given the
overall low incidence of a reaction; in fact, some have
advocated abandoning this procedure altogether (Tramer
et al. 2006). Patients with a history of severe contrast
allergy who will likely need IV contrast during a procedure should probably receive preexposure treatment with
corticosteroids (such as prednisone or hydrocortisone) as
well as H1 blockers—although strong evidence of benefit is lacking (Trcka et al. 2008). If contrast administration
cannot be delayed for four to six hours after steroids, some
would omit use and administer only H1 blockers (Royal

College of Radiologists 2010). Weaker agents—such as low-osmolar or iso-osmolar contrast such as ioxaglate, iohexol, or ioversol—should be used due to the lower overall incidence of reactions in patients with a history of asthma or a contrast allergy. The specific contrast agent causing the prior reaction should be sought and avoided if possible, although this information is often difficult for your doctor to obtain. Despite pretreatment with steroids and H1-blockers, reactions are still possible in those with prior reactions.

Thyroid Issues (Williams and Stevenson 2012). Hypothyroidism (low thyroid function) has been found in 0.5–0.8 percent of the population; it is demonstrated by elevated serum levels of thyroid-stimulating hormone (TSH) or decreased serum thyroxine levels (Murkin 1982). Undiagnosed (hence, untreated) hypothyroidism can lead to major perioperative complications including severe hypotension (low blood pressure) or cardiac arrest following induction of anesthesia, extreme sensitivity to narcotics and anesthetics with prolonged unconsciousness, and hypothyroid coma following anesthesia and surgery (Murkin 1982). Ideally, hypothyroidism is caught early in the preoperative evaluation, and thyroid supplement (thyroxine) may be administered until the patient's thyroid function has normalized—generally in four to six weeks.

Hyperthyroidism (high thyroid function) affects approximately 0.2 percent of men and 2 percent of women and may cause atrial fibrillation, congestive heart failure, and low blood cells (thrombocytopenia) (Farling 2000). In addition, anesthetic drugs may be affected by the hypermetabolic state of hyperthyroidism. When total intravenous anesthesia is used—often at our center this occurs when high-frequency ventilation is used to minimize respiratory motion during heart procedures—an increased dose of sedatives may be needed, because these agents are processed more quickly with a hyperactive thyroid (Farling 2000; Williams et al. 2011).

Generally, more thyroid-related perioperative complications stem from hypothyroidism as opposed to hyperthyroidism; however, recognition of either condition prior to implantation is important. Our Heart Rhythm Center generally obtains TSH prior to all device implantation, and we often allow four to six weeks for the patient to become euthyroid prior to proceeding with surgery. Emergent cases with thyroid abnormalities require close coordination with anesthesiology and will generally be undertaken with general anesthesia.

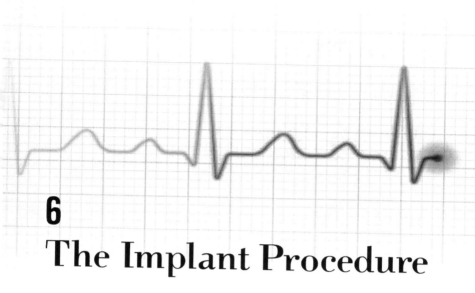

6
The Implant Procedure

Registration and check-in. Patients generally undergo defibrillator implantations at the hospital and require an overnight stay. Rarely do patients go home the same day as an implant procedure, although this can happen. Some doctors operate at multiple hospitals, so it is important to make sure at which hospital the procedure is to be done. The patients will generally check in with registration and then go to the appropriate *holding area* (pre-operative or "preop" unit). This is a staging area where the patient changes into a gown, an IV is started, and hospital documentation is performed. At this time, the patient is asked multiple times his or her name and the type of procedure that is to be performed. Questions often seem redundant—e.g., Do you have any allergies? What surgery are you here for?—but this fact-checking is an attempt to minimize any chance of medical error. Most implanting doctors will meet their patients here to answer any last-minute questions and confirm that all preoperative tests are complete and the surgery can proceed.

Informed-consent process. The informed-consent process is one of the most important aspects of any medical procedure. It is more than just getting a patient to sign the consent form. This is the process by which a patient is informed of the diagnosis and the nature and purpose of the proposed treatment or procedure. The patient should understand the risks and benefits of the proposed defibrillator implantation as well as the risks and benefits of any alternative treatments, such as medications or watchful waiting. Obviously, this book can be part of the informed-consent process, because it covers more thoroughly the entire defibrillator-implantation process than can be presented in even multiple office visits. It is during this process that patients can ask questions to be sure they fully understand the rationales for their defibrillators and can ask questions they might have for the physician. Some physicians go over these risks, benefits, and alternatives in the office and have their patients more thoroughly review and read the consent form at home prior to surgery. Once the patient has completed the required elements in the holding area and the informed-consent process is completed, he or she is brought into the *procedure room.*

The procedure room. The procedure room may be a standard operating room or may be a specialized cardiac-catheterization laboratory (where heart catheterizations are usually performed) that has been altered to perform defibrillator (and pacemaker) implantations. A *time-out* (once the patient is in the procedure room) occurs when the doctors, nurses, technologists, and all other personnel that are participating in the surgery stop what they are doing (before the patient is sedated) and identify the patient, the procedure being performed (including site of implant), the technique to be used, and any other important patient information (such as drug allergies). The time-out is performed to minimize the occurrence of any medical errors—like placing a defibrillator in the wrong patient!

At this point in time, the procedure can be started. Most patients are sedated for the defibrillator implantation. Conscious sedation involves giving medications that relax the patient and relieve pain but allow the patient to breathe on his or her own. Conscious sedation can be administered by nurses in the room or by anesthesiologists. General anesthesia involves deep sedation, and it often requires a temporary breathing tube and a connection to an artificial ventilator. General anesthesia is administered by anesthesiologists or specially trained nurses called *certified registered nurse anesthetists* (CRNAs). The higher the risk of the surgery, the more often general anesthesia is used. General anesthesia may permit tighter control of patient heart rate and blood pressure and allow the patient to remain absolutely still during the procedure. These elements may permit a safer procedure as well as a more pleasant experience for the patient.

The implant procedure. The implant procedure is performed under sterile conditions in an operating room or cardiac procedure room that includes sterile supplies, a patient table that is adjustable, and an x-ray system called fluoroscopy. Figure 9 shows a typical implant-procedure room. The C-arm holds the x-ray equipment that the physician uses to guide defibrillator leads into the correct positions; this technique of using x-rays to guide implantation is called fluoroscopy. The screens display patient information—like EKG and blood pressure—and show the x-ray images. The anesthesia equipment and anesthesiologist are at the head of the bed. A special sterile table holds all the instruments and equipment that will be used during the implantation.

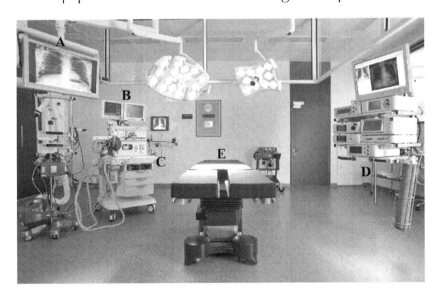

Figure 9. The Implant-Procedure Room. This is a dedicated implant-procedure room that includes (A) x-ray equipment to permit lead placement, (B) screens displaying patient information, (C) anesthesia equipment, (D) equipment to program the newly implanted defibrillator, and (E) the patient table.

THE IMPLANT PROCEDURE | **67**

The components of a defibrillator are described in chapter four. Most defibrillators are placed under the left collarbone. Most patients are right-handed, so left-sided implants are preferred. There are two reasons for this: 1) it is technically less demanding to place pacemaker leads from this location, and 2) any complications that occur are worse if they occur on the side of the patient's dominant arm. The most common access site is the left subclavian vein (or axillary vein). Often, more experienced implanters can perform a left-cephalic vein cutdown. This approach has been associated with fewer complications: such as pneumothorax, hemothorax, or lead fractures. I may attempt left-cephalic cut-down on patients at high risk of complications: such as extremely elderly patients (age greater than eighty years) or very small patients (weighing less than one hundred pounds). It is difficult to implant a device with more than one or two leads via a cephalic-cut-down approach due to the diminutive size of the cephalic vein.

The incision location is generally located two finger breadths below the clavicle. It is important to note that the ultimate location of the incision and device may vary considerably depending upon patient size. I may place an incision two finger breadths below the clavicle during the surgery, but when the patient wakes and stands up, he or she may see a considerable shift of the chest-wall tissue, which causes the device to be substantially lower. This shifting of the incision and defibrillator can be seen in both obese and thin patients.

Operative Steps of Defibrillator Implantation

1. Sterile preparation and draping of the patient occur on the operating table.

2. The patient is sedated.

3. Specialized personnel prepare the implant area under the right or left collarbone and cover the rest of the patient with sterile gowns.

4. The implanting physician sterilely scrubs hands for several minutes and then puts on a sterile gown and gloves.

5. Lidocaine is used to numb the skin, and a one- to three-inch incision is made.

6. A device pocket is made under the skin but above the chest-wall muscle. This pocket will hold the defibrillator and any extra lead material.

7. The subclavian vein is punctured with a needle, and a wire is placed through this needle. The needle is withdrawn—leaving the wire in the vein. Over this wire, a hollow tube is placed, and the defibrillator lead is placed through this hollow tube. Once the lead is attached to the heart, the hollow tube is removed, and the lead is sewn in place to the chest-wall muscle. This is repeated for each defibrillator lead.

8. The leads are tested to be sure they are functioning well and then are attached to the defibrillator. The defibrillator is then placed into the pocket with the leads coiled underneath. Defibrillation-threshold testing may be performed at this time.

9. The incision is then closed with several layers of sutures. The top layer of skin may be closed with staples or Steri-Strips™.

10. A sterile dressing is placed, and the patient is wakened from sedation and returned to the recovery area.

What happens if my doctor could not successfully place a left-ventricular lead? Placement of a pacing lead in the left ventricle via the coronary sinus can add time, complexity, and risk to a defibrillator implantation. It can be accomplished using the percutaneous technique (i.e., using the small incision in your upper chest and feeding the leads through veins) approximately 90 to 95 percent of the time. Unfortunately, a patient's anatomy may make it unfeasible to implant a lead at the time of initial defibrillator surgery. Your doctor may refer you to a heart surgeon to place the left-ventricular lead on the outside of your heart (the epicardium). This may require a staged (or multistep) procedure with a longer postoperative recovery due to the more complex surgery required to place the lead epicardially, that is, on the outside of your heart.

Immediately postimplant. Once the patient is awake with no obvious complications, he or she is generally observed in the hospital overnight though some centers may offer to send patients home the same day. Your doctor will usually talk to patient and family about the procedure. The discussion with family or friends is important; the patient may not remember events in the immediate postoperative period because of the sedatives given during the procedure. In our Heart Rhythm Center, patients are kept lying in bed for four hours after the implantation. They can eat once they are awake and alert after the procedure. We keep a sterile dressing on the wound until the next morning when we examine the incision. Some centers perform a chest x-ray immediately after the implantation. However, if the patient has had no obvious implant complications, I usually obtain a chest x-ray (CXR) the next morning to verify that the leads are still in the correct position. A typical postimplant CXR is shown in figure 10. We use this postimplant chest x-ray to verify correct lead position and assess for complications. I have included an overlay of the heart's anatomy to give you an idea of heart-chamber locations.

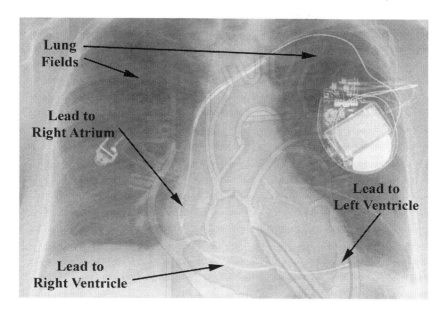

Lung Fields

Lead to Right Atrium

Lead to Left Ventricle

Lead to Right Ventricle

Figure 10. The Basics of Reading a Chest X-Ray. This is a typical postimplant chest x-ray—with a superimposed cartoon of the heart to show you *approximate* location of cardiac chambers—used to verify correct lead position and assess for complications. Your cardiologist uses the CXR to make sure that the leads are in the correct chamber of the heart. We normally look for damage to the lungs and lead positions after the implant is completed.

Day after the implantation. The morning after the implantation, the sterile dressing is removed and the incision is inspected by the doctor, nurse, or an assistant. I commonly leave a layer of butterfly stiches (Steri-Strips™) over the incision. Generally, the incision can be left without a gauze dressing—as long as the incision-care instructions in next section are followed. If there is any oozing, clean, dry gauze can be placed over the incision to protect clothing from blood staining. Finally, the device is *interrogated*, using a special bedside computer called a *programmer.* Figure 11 shows a mock interrogation being performed. Usually an electronic wand is placed over the pacemaker site, and it is used to exchange information with the defibrillator. The programmer is used to check the lead functions and send any programming changes to the defibrillator. Generally, patients do not feel any symptoms during device checks and programming, but a patient can occasionally notice different heart rates during the check. Once the defibrillator is interrogated, any changes are saved onto the defibrillator, and the patient is ready to go home. The implanting physician may not see the patient the day after implantation, but the physician's team will be very familiar with device care and the process of arranging postimplant discharge from the hospital.

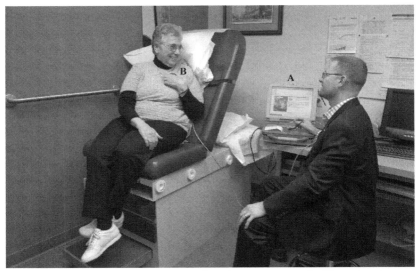

Figure 11. Device Interrogation. This shows a typical office visit for a defibrillator check (called *interrogation*). The programmer A) has all the software necessary to check and program the defibrillator. Many

defibrillators allow wireless interrogations, but many still require a wand B) that is held over the defibrillator to communicate with the device.

What is defibrillator-threshold testing (DFT)? Defibrillator-threshold tests are performed at the end of a defibrillator-implant surgery. Through DFTs we check to make sure a defibrillator can effectively detect and treat ventricular fibrillation. I always find it very difficult to explain this to patients in a single office visit where I also have to learn all their past medical history and explain the process of implantation as well as the recovery process. We implant the defibrillator to immediately treat a VT/VF cardiac arrest, so it intuitively (to me) makes sense that we would want to cause VT/VF (in the controlled situation of the operating room) and make sure the device can detect it and terminate it. Believe it or not, this is generally well tolerated by the patient, and it results in no complications. There is a very small risk of sustained VT/VF that cannot be terminated by our traditional means in the operating room.

What does it mean if you fail DFTs? Sometimes the implanted defibrillator does not have enough power (energy) to terminate the VT/VF. In this case, we usually then resort to externally applied defibrillator pads to terminate the VT/VF. We can often program the defibrillator to better treat VT/VF, and sometimes we have to add special leads (subcutaneous arrays or azygous/coronary-sinus coils) that permit a more effective energy delivery.

What if my doctor doesn't perform DFTs? Sometimes there may be other medical reasons for your doctor to not perform DFTs. These conditions include but are not limited to: intracardiac thrombi (blood clots in your heart), atrial fibrillation, significant heart-valve disease, low blood pressures, severe coronary blockages that cannot be fixed, recent heart attack or stroke, or morbid obesity. Current defibrillators have become so good that DFTs may not be mandatory if the patient has one of these conditions.

When is it necessary to perform DFTs with an existing defibrillator? A patient that could not undergo DFTs at the initial implantation may be brought back several weeks/months after the surgery to do so. Sometimes, new medications are started that may affect the ability of a device to deliver an effective therapy. The most common medication that can affect DFTs is amiodarone. This medicine is given to patients to prevent atrial- and ventricular-rhythm abnormalities.

Talk to your doctor about any questions you have about DFTs.

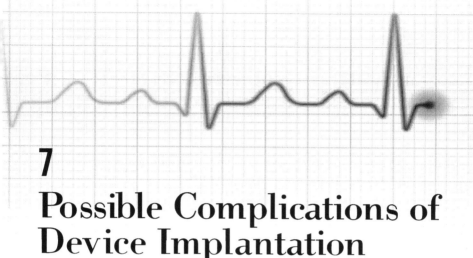

7
Possible Complications of Device Implantation

Introduction. This section is written for both patients and primary-care doctors, even though it is a bit more complex than the rest of the book. In most cases, I have attempted to boil the complication rates down to simple percentages and show the imaging that I use to detect these complications. It will familiarize patients with the names of common complications and how we detect and treat them. I strived to provide the best image of a particular complication; in some cases, the device pictured is a pacemaker rather than a defibrillator. In addition, it is heavily referenced to demonstrate the basis for the estimated rate of complications and provide physicians with further reading material. For a more detailed discussion on complications of device implantation that

Dr. Robert Stevenson and I coauthored, please see: http://www.intechopen.com/books/current-issues-and-recent-advances-in-pacemaker-therapy/complications_of_pacemaker_implantation (Williams and Stevenson 2012).

Major and minor complications can occur in approximately 4 to 8 percent of patients within six weeks of defibrillator implantation (Bristow et al. 2004; Alter et al. 2005; Bardy et al. 2005; Moss et al. 2009; Williams and Stevenson 2012). This means that for every one hundred patients who undergo a defibrillator implantation, four to eight patients may experience a major or minor complication. Depending on the implanting physician, these rates of major and minor complications can be as high as 10 to 15 percent within six weeks of a defibrillator implantation. Keep in mind this includes both major *and* minor complications added together. Furthermore, most defibrillator implantations are performed on an elective, outpatient basis. We generally find that complications (and hospital readmissions) tend to occur more frequently in patients who are admitted to the hospital for other reasons (such as heart attacks, cardiac arrests, and chronic pulmonary or kidney issues; Reynolds 2006) and undergo a defibrillator implant during that hospitalization.

Figure 12 shows the incidence of specific types of complications that can occur during pacemaker implantation; I use pacemakers as an example because there tend to be more detailed data available on pacemaker-implant complications. The diamond shows the average rate that the complication occurs as a percentage; the bars depict the range of complication rates that is possible. For instance, leads become dislodged an average of 2.3 percent of the time as reported in prior trials, although it can vary from 0.5 to 4 percent of the time—depending upon the implanting physician. The rates of complications for defibrillators tend to be slightly higher than pacemaker implants due to the increased complexity of these devices. We also tend to see a higher rate of complications in women and minorities (Reynolds 2006). A real-world look at defibrillator implantations estimates a 0.8 to 1.7 percent death rate associated with defibrillator implantation (Ezekowitz et al. 2007). In addition, the more complex the device (e.g., three leads versus only one lead), the more likely a possible complication will occur. Complications have important patient-care implications, but they also increase the hospitalization cost and postoperative length of stay. Moreover, patients who experience a major complication have an increased risk of death (three to fourfold increase; Lee 2010) up to six months after defibrillator implantation!

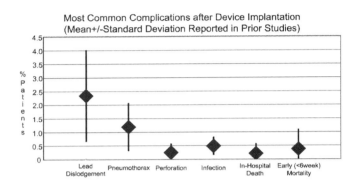

Figure 12. Most Common Complications after Device Implantation
(Figure originally published by Williams and Stevenson 2012)

Major complications have been defined as death, cardiac arrest, cardiac perforation, cardiac-valve injury, coronary-venous dissection, hemothorax, pneumothorax, transient ischemic attack, stroke, myocardial infarction, pericardial tamponade, and arterial-venous fistula. Minor complications have been defined as drug reaction, conduction block, hematoma or lead dislodgement requiring reoperation, peripheral embolus, phlebitis, peripheral nerve injury, and device-related infection. One of the major techniques we use to evaluate for complications from defibrillator implantation is the chest x-ray (also called chest radiograph). Figure 10 (in chapter 6) shows a typical chest x-ray of a patient after undergoing a defibrillator implantation. The defibrillator device is placed in the left-upper chest, and leads are seen in the right atrium, right ventricle, and left ventricle (via the coronary sinus). One can see the lung fields, cardiac silhouette, ribs, and diaphragm. The chest x-ray can be quickly assessed for lead position and damage to the heart or lungs.

There is obviously a difference in complication rates based upon the operating physician and the hospital in which the physician practices. I examined the complication rates of the first consecutive 250 device implants performed when starting a new electrophysiology program at a community hospital (Williams et al. 2010). Figure 13 shows complication rates of device implantation of our program (blue dots) versus those at non–community hospitals (blocks and stripes). I did not have any major complications in this series of patients; however, I have had major complications for defibrillator implantations. It is important to note that past success rates do not guarantee future performance. All procedures have a risk of complications! See chapter 5 for the questions to ask your doctor before having surgery.

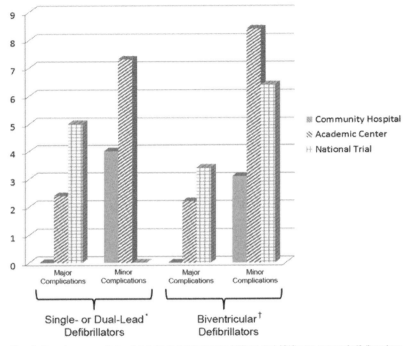

Figure 13. Device-Implantation Complication Rates in Various Hospital Settings

Complications that can occur prior to going home.

Sedation/Airway: Less than 20 percent of electrophysiology (EP) programs in the United States exclusively use anesthesia professionals for procedural sedation (Gaitan 2011). Minor complications (e.g., atelectasis or minor lung compression, fever, or vascular congestion) may simply be reflective of the common, postoperative pulmonary complications (PPC) seen after general anesthesia. Atelectasis can be seen on CT scan in up to 90 percent of patients who are anesthetized (Magnusson and Spahn 2003) and PPCs have been found to occur in 9.6 percent of patients (Lawrence et al. 1995). There are data to suggest that patients undergoing invasive EP procedures may require deep-conscious sedation that often is converted to general anesthesia (Trentman et al. 2009); thus, the use of general anesthesia (including high-frequency ventilation to minimize patient movement) during EP procedures may enhance patient safety (DiBiase et al. 2011; Williams et al. 2011).

Pneumothorax: Pneumothorax may occur in as many as 3 to 4 percent (Hargreaves, Doulalas, and Ormerod 1995; Noseworthy et al. 2004) and as few as 0 to 1 percent (Williams and Stevenson 2012; Williams et al. 2010) but generally ranges from 1 to 3 percent of patients undergoing device implantation (Parsonnet, Bernstein, and Lindsay 1989; Link et al. 1998; Ellenbogen 2003). A pneumothorax is a collection of air outside the lung but underneath the lung lining (pleural space). It can cause the lung to collapse. It is caused by damaging the lung during lead placement and is often more common in smokers or extremely thin patients. Routine chest radiographs may be performed immediately after defibrillator implantation, and clinical signs of pneumothorax include low oxygen on pulse oximetry, shortness of breath, pleuritic pain (pain that is worse with deep breathing), and low blood pressure. Figure 14 depicts the radiographic appearance of small, medium, and large pneumothoraces. Emergent treatment of pneumothorax includes decompression of the pressure built up by the air collection. This decompression is done by placing a tube through the chest wall to drain the air collection (called *pleurocentesis*). This can be done by the implanting physician, but it is usually performed by a surgeon. Often, high concentrations of inspired oxygen can lead to a resolution of a small pneumothorax (comprising less than 30 percent lung volume; Chadha and Cohn 1983). This conservative treatment of pneumothorax can reduce further complications and duration of hospitalization and avoid invasive drainage procedures. The traditional treatment of patients with traumatic (e.g., motor-vehicle accidents) hemothoraces or pneumothoraces has been an insertion of a chest tube (CT). Chest tubes have larger caliber than smaller pigtail catheters and can cause significant trauma during insertion, cause pain, prevent full lung expansion, and worsen pulmonary outcomes (Kulvatunyou 2011). Pigtail catheters—smaller and less invasive than chest tubes—have been used successfully in patients with nontraumatic pneumothorax (e.g., those occurring during defibrillator implantation).

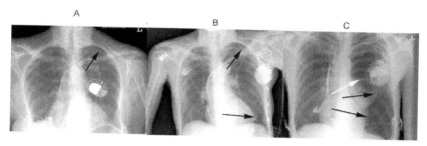

Figure 14. Examples of Pneumothoraces, Small (A), Medium (B), and Large (C). The edge of the pneumothorax is indicated by the arrows. A small left apical pneumothorax is shown in A. A medium-sized apical and basilar pneumothorax is shown in B. An almost complete collapse of the left lung is shown in C. Please note that the example shown in A is from a pacemaker implantation. (Figure originally published by Williams and Stevenson 2012)

Vascular access and bleeding (Hemothorax): The axillary axillary-venous approach has been associated with less frequent pneumothorax and subclavian-crush syndrome (damage to the vein that can cause the arm to swell; Fyke 1993; Magney et al. 1993). The axillary vein is the continuation of the basilica vein—it runs over the bicep muscle in the arm—that terminates immediately beneath the collar bone at the outer border of the first rib, at which point it becomes the subclavian vein (Belott 2006). Direct subclavian venous punctures are associated with increased rate of pneumothorax (Chadha and Cohn 1983) while cephalic-vein cut-down has been associated with the lowest rate of pneumothorax and lead damage (Parsonnet, Bernstein, and Lindsay 1989; Williams and Stevenson 2012).

Fluoroscopic-guided, first-rib approach to axillary-vein access is the most effective means to access the vessel while minimizing the risk of pneumothorax (Belott 2006). The cephalic-vein cut-down is an advanced technique that allows us to place device wires without poking a needle in the patient's chest wall; not all implanting physicians can perform this technique, so check with your implanting physician to see if this is an option. Furthermore, the cephalic vein in small patients may not be large enough to implant multiple defibrillator leads.

Hemothorax (bleeding into the rib cage around the lungs) can be caused by lead placement (more frequently atrial-lead perforation) as well as vascular-access damage to the subclavian and axillary veins and the vena cava. A prior study examined device implantation complication rates of 632 consecutive implants at a single noncommunity institution (Chadha and Cohn 1983). They found a 0.6 percent rate of hemothorax with a substantially large incidence of complications experienced by low-volume (fewer than twelve implants per year) implanters. Figure 15 depicts a postimplant CXR of a hemothorax occurring during upgrade of dual-chamber pacemaker to biventricular defibrillator. Recognition of new effusions should be treated as possible procedure-related hemothorax, and surgical consultation may be warranted.

A

B

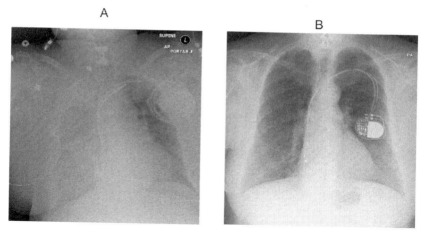

Figure 15. Hemothorax after Device Implantation. The right hemithorax has a layered effusion with blunting of the right diaphragm (hazy portion on left side of image A). Image B depicts the preoperative radiograph prior to upgrade of pacemaker to defibrillator. (Figure originally published by Williams and Stevenson 2012)

It is important to ask your doctor the type of implant technique he or she uses. Again, an important question to ask is this: how many devices has he or she implanted? No matter what vascular-access technique used, generally, the more experience a doctor has, the lower the complication rate.

Perforation/Tamponade. Perforation occurs when trauma causes an unintended hole in a blood vessel or the walls of the heart; it can be a life-threatening situation. Perforation (both acute and subacute) has been reported to occur in up to 1 percent of device implantations (Williams and Stevenson 2012; Williams et al. 2010;

Ellenbogen 2003; Link et al. 1998; Reynolds 2006). In addition, asymptomatic subclinical (does not cause worrisome symptoms) perforation may occur in 15 percent of patients after device implantation (Hirschl et al. 2007). Symptoms of perforation include: pleuritic chest pain from pericarditis, diaphragmatic- or intercostal-muscle stimulation (which feels like involuntary and sometimes painful hiccups), and, in the presence of pericardial effusion (blood collecting around the outside of the heart), the possible development of shortness of breath and hypotension as tamponade develops (Wang et al. 2009). Tamponade occurs when enough blood collects on the outside of the heart that it can compress the heart and render it unable to pump blood effectively. Other signs/ symptoms of perforation include EKG abnormalities or friction rub (which sounds like rubbing sandpaper heard on stethoscope) after implant. If perforation is suspected, urgent evaluation of the patient and device function is warranted, though lead parameters are often within normal limits (Wang et al. 2009).

Figure 16 shows examples of coronary-sinus damage that can occur during LV-lead implantation. Figure 17 depicts right-ventricular lead perforations. Cardiac surgery is typically not required for a majority of patients diagnosed with cardiac perforation from a defibrillator implantation. Rather, most cases can be managed with pericardiocentesis (drainage of blood with a small catheter) performed by an interventional cardiologist for symptomatic effusions and by repositioning of the lead in the EP laboratory with close cardiothoracic surgical collaboration (Wang et al. 2009; Mahapatra 2005; Geyfman et al. 2007). Figure 18 shows a large cardiac silhouette—developing after pacemaker implantation—that was due to large pericardial effusion. The effusion was treated with pericardiocentesis (with no evidence of blood reaccumulation) and did not require lead repositioning. Though perforation and subsequent tamponade are infrequent complications of device implantation, they can be responsible for significant patient morbidity (any untoward side effect from a procedure) and mortality (death). The risks of perforation cannot be underestimated; death from tamponade with subsequent cardiac arrest was responsible for 21.8 percent of the deaths in a worldwide study of perforation after ablation for atrial fibrillation (Cappato et al. 2009). There is some evidence that passive-fixation leads cause fewer ventricular perforations, because there is no screw at the tip of the lead. The selection of passive versus active fixation involves many factors, such as patient anatomy, risk of complications, and implanter experience. It is important to ask your doctor what leads he or she will be using for your defibrillator—and why. Passive-fixation leads are much more common with pacemakers rather than defibrillators.

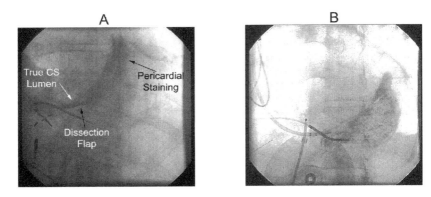

Figure 16. Damage to the Coronary Sinus during Left-Ventricular-Lead Implantation. Image A depicts a dissection/perforation flap and the resulting pericardial staining from engaging the coronary sinus with a deflectable electrophysiology-recording catheter. Image B shows a similar instance of pericardial staining with no focal dissection flap or perforation. Both patients underwent successful LV-lead implantation at the time. (Figure originally published by Williams and Stevenson 2012)

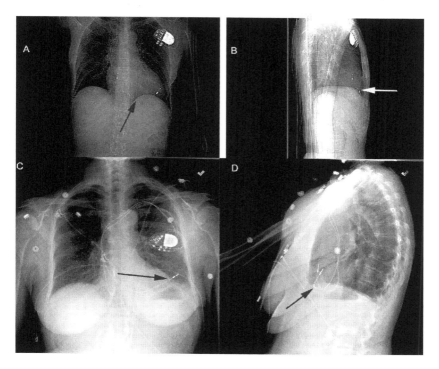

Figure 17. Examples of Right-Ventricular Lead Perforation. Images A and B depict an RV-lead perforation that exits the right-ventricular base in A (arrow) and reenters near the right-ventricular apex in B (arrow). Images C and D depict a right-ventricular apical perforation. The lead is seen exiting the cardiac silhouette in C (arrow); the lateral view (D) depicts an abrupt change in lead course (arrow) that is often seen in right-ventricular apical perforations as the lead courses posteriorly in the pericardial space. (Figure originally published by Williams and Stevenson 2012)

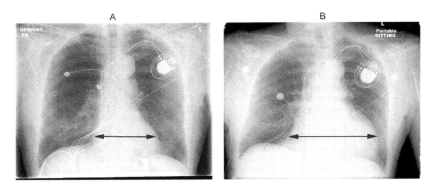

Figure 18. Chest Radiograph Appearance of Large Pericardial Effusion after RV-Lead Perforation. Immediate postimplant CXR (A) shows normal appearance of the cardiac silhouette. Two weeks postoperative CXR performed, because patient-reported symptoms of chest pressure (B) shows enlarged cardiac silhouette. Patient responded to pericardiocentesis with no lead repositioning. (Figure originally published by Williams and Stevenson 2012)

Complications of left-ventricular (LV) lead placement via the coronary sinus. Resynchronization devices (biventricular defibrillators) are often used for patients with heart failure by placing a pacing lead in the left ventricle to "resynchronize" the pumping action of the heart so that the right and left ventricles pump at the same time. The emergence of resynchronization therapy has led to an increase in attempts at LV-lead placement via the coronary sinus. The MIRACLE study program (Leon et al. 2005) reported a 91.6 percent success rate for LV-lead placement, while COMPANION (Bristow et al. 2004) revealed an 89 percent success rate for LV-lead placement. Another report indicated a similar 92 percent success rate with LV-lead placement (D'Ivernois, Lesage, and Blanc 2008). Though I counsel my patients on an LV-lead placement success rate at 90 to 95 percent, we have demonstrated a 97 percent success rate (sixty-four of sixty-six patients) with LV-lead placement within the range from 2:30 to 5:30 o'clock in the left-anterior-oblique (LAO) view (Williams et al. 2010).

Complications of LV-lead placement include: cardiac perforation (poking hole in wall of vessel), coronary-sinus dissection (damaging the vessel wall), electrical trauma (heart block), failure to place the lead, dislodgement of the lead, and diaphragmatic stimulation (Ellery and Paul 2004). Coronary-sinus dissections or perforations, cardiac perforations, or cardiac-vein dissections or perforations were reported in 45 of 2078 cases (2 percent) in the MIRACLE study program (Leon et al. 2005). Figure 16 depicts damage that can be done to the coronary sinus during LV-lead implantation.

Loss of LV capture (the lead cannot pace) and diaphragmatic stimulation leading to interruption of resynchronization therapy have been found to occur in 10 percent and 2 percent of patients, respectively (Knight et al. 2004). Diaphragmatic stimulation occurs when the pacing lead is placed too close to the phrenic nerve and can actually pace the diaphragm; this may occur in up to 5 to 10 percent of patients. This diaphragmatic pacing is not dangerous, but it can be uncomfortable; it feels like a "grabbing" or hiccup in the left chest or rib cage. The development of new LV leads (with up to four electrodes) offers the possibility of numerous pacing locations that can minimize loss of capture and diaphragmatic stimulation.

Arrhythmias (supraventricular tachycardia, ventricular tachycardia, ventricular fibrillation). The incidence of sustained atrial, pacemaker-mediated, and ventricular-rhythm disturbances from device implantation is low (Jordaens 1989). In patients without prior atrial arrhythmias, Jordaens et al. found early atrial fibrillation (during the first week after implantation) in 2 of 112 patients, late atrial fibrillation in 7 patients, and atrial flutter in 1, yielding a total incidence of 8.9 percent for 22 months. There were no significant differences with respect to age, etiology (cause), electrocardiographic diagnosis, pacing history, or the measured intracardiac P wave between the group with and the group without atrial fibrillation. Ventricular fibrillation has been reported to occur in 0.1 percent of all patients undergoing pacemaker implantation and up to 0.6 percent of patients aged greater than ninety years undergoing pacemaker implantation (Williams and Stevenson 2012).

It has been reported that ventricular tachyarrhythmias (e.g., ventricular tachycardia or fibrillation) may be present in 12 to 31 percent of patients months to years after device implantation (Faber et al. 2007), but this may reflect underlying progression of heart disease. However, there are several situations where device leads and pacing may cause the abnormal ventricular arrhythmias. These include device-lead irritation of the right-ventricular inflow (Datta et al. 2011) and outflow tracts (Bohm et al. 2002), pacemaker stimulus on T wave (Freedman et al. 1982), reentrant circuit around endocardial-device lead (Li, Sarubbi, and Somerville 2000) and bradycardia-dependent VT facilitated by long pause caused by myopotential inhibition of a single-chamber (ventricular lead) device (Iesaka et al. 1982). As true with most other device-related implant complications, there is a slightly higher incidence of arrhythmias after defibrillator implantation. Up to 8 percent of patients may experience a worsening of ventricular tachycardia or new-onset atrial fibrillation after a defibrillator implantation (Ong 1995). There is a higher incidence of arrhythmias if patients had leads placed epicardially (on the outside of the heart).

Heart attacks. Heart attacks are also called *myocardial infarctions* (MIs) and are the most common cause of death after any surgery. They generally occur in less than 1 percent of defibrillator surgeries. Again, the implanting physician generally assesses the risk of surgery prior to the procedure, and patients at high risk of heart attacks may need additional heart care prior to proceeding with defibrillator implantation. *Keep in mind—the very patients who have advanced coronary-artery disease causing heart failure can be at the highest risk for perioperative heart attacks.*

Death. In-hospital death generally occurs in less than 1 percent of device implantations (Williams and Stevenson 2012; Link et al. 1998; Reynolds 2006); however, there is a concern that death is underreported, because some studies do not specifically mention perioperative death (Parsonnet, Bernstein, and Lindsay 1989; Williams and Stevenson 2012). The most common causes of confirmed device-related in-hospital deaths are perforations of the subclavian artery, brachiocephalic trunk, right atrium, and right ventricle. The most common cause of non-device-related in-hospital death is myocardial infarction (heart attack) as well as, less commonly, pulmonary embolism, stroke, heart failure, and sepsis (Schulza, Puschelb, and Turkc 2009).

Pocket hematoma. A pocket hematoma is a collection of blood around the device but underneath the skin. Figure 19F shows an example of a pocket hematoma. The incidence of pocket hematoma has been reported at 4.9 percent and leading to prolonged hospitalization in 2.0 percent of all patients (Wiegand et al. 2004). Reoperation for pocket hematoma—to drain the collection of blood—may occur in up to 1.0 percent of patients. An informal look at our Heart Rhythm Center outcomes revealed no reoperations for hematomas in our first 1275 device implants. High-dose heparinization, combined acetylsalicylic acid (ASA or aspirin)/thienopyridine (such as clopidogrel, Plavix®) treatment after coronary stenting, and low operator experience were independently predictive of hematoma development (Wiegand et al. 2004). In addition, *development of postoperative hematoma places the patient at elevated risk of device infection* (Sohail et al. 2011). Most hematomas resolve with watchful waiting and do not require a repeat surgery. They resolve over four to six weeks and can often have significant associated bruising, which also resolves over that time period. Worrisome signs include continued swelling, redness, warmth, bleeding, oozing, or changes in the incision. It is important to call the implanting physician with any worries about incision or pocket healing.

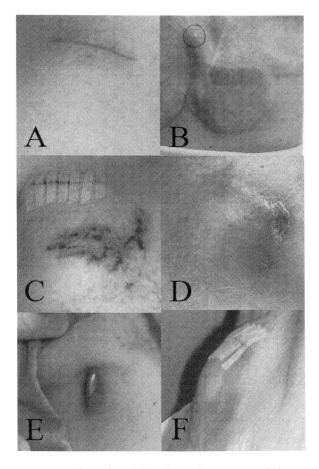

Figure 19A–F. Examples of Incisional Healing. Normal device pocket (A) several weeks after implantation shows a uniform incision and mild fullness representing the defibrillator in the pocket. Pocket and incisional thinning with prominent skin tenting from a lead (circle) in an extremely elderly patient is shown in (B). Redness and irritation from adhesive tape is shown in (C). One can see redness and skin breakdown seen with imminent erosion (D) that can lead to complete erosion (breaks through the skin) of the defibrillator (E). Finally, (F) depicts a pocket hematoma.

There is data to suggest that warfarin (Coumadin®) causes fewer pocket complications than heparin products. Specifically, temporarily interrupting anticoagulation (e.g., stopping Coumadin) is associated with increased thromboembolic events (e.g., strokes or transient ischemic attacks), whereas cessation of warfarin with bridging anticoagulation with heparin products is associated with a higher rate of pocket hematoma and a longer hospital stay (Ahmed et al. 2010). The issue of perioperative anticoagulation is very important to discuss with the doctor who will be performing the defibrillator implantation. I routinely perform device implants while continuing warfarin uninterrupted.

Lengths of hospital stay: A large study looked at over thirty thousand Medicare patients who underwent defibrillator implantation, and it found an average post–defibrillator-implant length of hospital stay of four to five days (Reynolds 2006). Our experience with 250 consecutive device implantations (Williams et al. 2010) revealed an average length of postimplant hospital stay of two to three days; however, over 90 percent of generator changes (for example, no new leads were implanted and only the defibrillator can was replaced) were discharged home the same day. There is evidence that complications cause a substantial increase in the length of stay up to sixteen days (Ferguson et al. 1996). The mean costs of complications are as follows: $4345 ± $1540 for device-lead revision, $24,459 ± $14,585 for device infection, and $6187 ± $2631 for hematoma evacuation (Ferguson et al. 1996).

POSSIBLE COMPLICATIONS OF DEVICE IMPLANTATION | **97**

Complications that usually occur within thirty days of implant. Only a small proportion of complications occur before going home after the defibrillator implantation (Lee 2010). This makes follow-up with your care providers (and ideally the implanting physician) very important.

Defibrillator and lead function/failures. Electrocardiographic signs of defibrillator-pacing malfunction can be grouped into four categories: failure to pace the heart, failure to deliver a pacing signal, undersensing, and inappropriate pacemaker rate. There is an overall device and lead malfunction rate in 1 to 3 percent of patients (Hayes and Vlietstra 1993).

Failure to pace the heart (loss of capture). Failure to pace the heart means that a pacing signal is delivered but does not result in a heartbeat. You may not even notice this occurring, but patients can often feel palpitations or dizziness, or they may even faint as a result. Loss of capture after defibrillator implantation (in a patient who requires pacing support) has many causes:

- *Dislodgement*: Lead has fallen out of place and likely is in an area that does not pace correctly.
- *Elevated thresholds*: Device requires more energy than normal to pace, which may lead to early battery depletion.
- *Inappropriate lead placement*: Lead may not be properly located and misplacement not discovered until follow-up.

- *Lead fracture*: Lead may break, very rarely and usually near the insertion site to the defibrillator header.
- *Insulation failure*: The silicone/plastic outer coating of the lead (insulator) has a defect and can cause the lead to malfunction.
- *Loose-set screw*: The screw that holds the lead in the defibrillator header may become loose.
- *Exit block (greater than four weeks)*: Scar formation developing at the tip of the lead where it contacts the heart makes pacing more difficult.
- *Perforation*: The leads poke through the wall of the heart, which may lead to bleeding or more serious complications.
- *Battery/circuit failure*: Very rare, and discussed in chapter 11.
- *Air in pocket*: During surgery, some air may remain in pocket and at times can cause issues until it is reabsorbed, over several weeks.
- *Metabolic/drugs (Flecainide)*: Medications and some illnesses can make it difficult for the lead to pace the heart.

Lead dislodgement, the most common cause of failure to capture (Hayes and Vlietstra 1993), has been reported to occur in up to 4 to 6 percent of device implantations (Reynolds 2006) but is generally reported with a 1 to 3 percent incidence (Williams and Stevenson 2012; Williams et al. 2010; Ellenbogen 2003; Link et al. 1998). Many patients have lead dislodgements within several hours of the implant surgery, but some lead dislodgments occur after they are sent home. Figures 20 and 21 depict examples of right-atrial-, right-ventricular-, and left-ventricular-lead dislodgements that may result in failure to pace the heart. Lead dislodgements are treated by repositioning the lead in the implant-procedure room. The LV lead has been found to dislodge more frequently than right-atrial and right-ventricular leads; LV-lead dislodgment may occur in between 3 to 10 percent of patients undergoing biventricular defibrillator implantations (van Rees et al. 2011). Dislodgment may result when a patient does not follow activity limitations after an implant or "twiddles" the device. Patients may also experience lead dislodgement through no fault of their own.

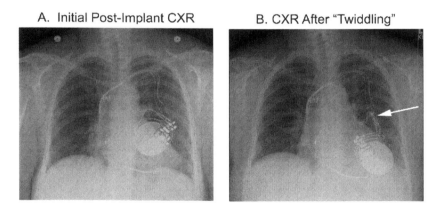

Figure 20. Lead Orientation before and after Patient Twiddling Resulted in Lead Dislodgement. *Twiddling* refers to patient manipulation of a defibrillator's can or leads, which may lead to malfunction. Image A depicts the postimplant-radiograph baseline lead positioning after biventricular defibrillator implant. Image B shows retracted right- and left-ventricular leads and leads tangled in the pocket superior to a device can that has been rotated by twiddling. (Figure originally published by Williams and Stevenson 2012)

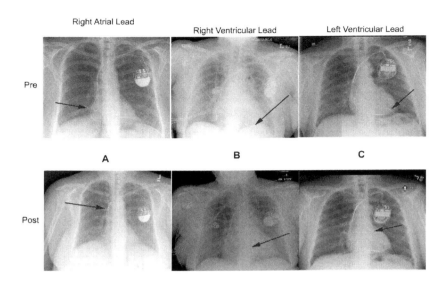

Figure 21. Right-Atrial (A), Right-Ventricular (B), and Left-Ventricular (C) Leads before (Pre) and after (Post) Dislodgements. Right-atrial lead became dislodged after patient twiddled with device. Right-ventricular lead dislodged by moving more basilar in position (arrow) one day after implant. Left-ventricular lead dislodged and reseated itself in the body of coronary sinus three months after initial placement (arrow; figure originally published by Williams and Stevenson 2012).

Failure to output: Failure of the device to deliver a pacing signal may be caused by battery or circuit failure, lead fracture, internal-insulation failure, oversensing, loose-set screw, or crosstalk. Complete device failure (due to a random component failure) is quite rare; however, total battery depletion can occur if routine device follow-up is inadequate (Hayes and Vlietstra 1993). Once initial battery end-of-life indicators appear, there is usually a period of months before the battery reaches a critically low voltage, and pacing and capability to deliver a lifesaving shock fails (Hayes and Vlietstra 1993). We usually estimate that once a defibrillator reaches the Elective Replacement Indicator, the patient can still get three months of pacing support (if need be) or ten defibrillator shocks before the battery is completely depleted.

The incidence of device-lead fracture (e.g., the lead breaks) has been reported at 0.1–4.2 percent per patient-year and usually occurs adjacent to the generator or near the site of venous access (Alt et al. 1987). Other electrical signals may cause noise and subsequent "oversensing" (and fool the defibrillator into inappropriately shocking the patient); commonly, the diaphragm's contracting can cause electrical signals (myopotentials) to be detected by the defibrillator (oversensing) and misinterpreted by the defibrillator (as a potentially fatal arrhythmia resulting in inappropriate therapy). Also, other sources of external electrical noise can affect device function (discussed in chapter 8).

Undersensing: Undersensing of intrinsic heartbeats results in inappropriate pacing output that competes with your native heartbeat. Undersensing is most likely caused by lead dislodgement, poor lead position at time of implantation, or an interruption in the insulation of the pacing lead (Hayes and Vlietstra 1993). Furthermore, undersensing may prevent your defibrillator from recognizing a potentially fatal heart rhythm.

Inappropriate pacemaker rate: There are several causes of inappropriate pacemaker rate, but most are not due to device malfunction except "runaway pacemaker." A "runaway pacemaker" is a true device failure that can rarely be caused by battery depletion, random component failure, or radiation treatments for cancer (Hayes and Vlietstra 1993). The more common causes of inappropriate pacing rate are not actual malfunctions of the device but issues that can be corrected by altering the defibrillator's programming. Pacing can be too slow if the device is oversensing or too fast if the device is undersensing. See above for descriptions of oversensing and undersensing.

Inappropriate Shocks or Therapy: Defibrillators have saved countless lives, but they are not foolproof. It is possible that the device can deliver unnecessary pacing (called *antitachycardia pacing*) or worse deliver an unnecessary shock. If this shock occurs while a patient is awake, it can be very painful. It is estimated that 5 to 20 percent of defibrillator patients receive inappropriate shocks (Ezekowitz et al. 2007). Inappropriate shocks happen because the defibrillator misinterprets external electrical signals (like noise from poorly grounded power tools) as the onset of a potentially fatal arrhythmia and treats it with an inappropriate therapy. See chapters 9 and 10 for what to do if you or your loved one receives a defibrillator shock.

Diaphragmatic Stimulation: Diaphragmatic stimulation occurs when the pacing lead (usually the left-ventricular lead) is placed too close to the phrenic nerve and actually paces the diaphragm. I rarely see it associated with a right-atrial or ventricular lead. This diaphragmatic pacing is usually not dangerous, but it can be uncomfortable; it feels like a "grabbing" or hiccup in the left chest or rib cage. Diaphragmatic stimulation can occur in up to 5 to 10 percent of patients. The development of new LV leads with up to four electrodes offers the possibility of numerous pacing locations that can minimize loss of capture and diaphragmatic stimulation. I often encounter this immediately after the implant, but it can often occur weeks to months after an implant. We can often reprogram the device to avoid diaphragmatic stimulation. Call your doctor should you have any new or concerning symptoms after a defibrillator implant.

Hospital readmission: We found that the average rate of readmission within six weeks of defibrillator implantation at our community hospital was 4.4 percent; of those, the majority of these readmissions were not device related or due to heart issues (Williams et al. 2010). Furthermore, we have found that patients undergoing device implantation already admitted to the hospital for other reasons (e.g., atrial fibrillation or heart failure) have higher rates of readmission than patients undergoing elective, outpatient device implantation. In the MADIT CRT study looking at biventricular defibrillators, approximately one in five patients were readmitted to the hospital for heart failure within two years of device implantation. Many (if not most) patients undergoing defibrillator implantation have heart failure and these patients have higher readmission rates than patients without heart failure.

There are many factors that can increase the likelihood of readmission to the hospital after a defibrillator implantation. Increased age and increased device complexity (e.g., generator changes that do not involve placement of new pacemaker leads are less complex than devices that require multiple new lead placements) may increase readmission rate (Williams and Stevenson 2012; Stevenson et al. 2012). Other factors that can increase risk of readmission include abnormal kidney function, emergency situation/presentation, ejection fraction, female gender, and small stature (weight less than one hundred pounds). Reasons for readmission are quite varied, but many result from the aforementioned complications in addition to heart failure, pneumonia, or strokes. Of note, the vast majority of patients who require defibrillators are aged greater than sixty-five years and often have other medical conditions that may be exacerbated by any surgical procedure.

Strokes: Strokes (also called *transient ischemic attacks* or *TIAs*) may occur immediately postoperatively or can occur several weeks out from implantation. Strokes generally occur in less than 1 percent of patients but have been seen in up to 1.4 percent of extremely elderly (age greater than eighty years) patients undergoing device implantation (Stevenson et al. 2012). I have most commonly seen strokes in patients who had anticoagulation (warfarin or Coumadin©) held temporarily for the surgery; the strokes occur during the time the anticoagulation was held until the patient has been effectively reanticoagulated after the surgery. There is data to suggest that device implantation can be safely performed without stopping warfarin and may lead to fewer complications (Ahmed et al. 2010). It is important to discuss management of anticoagulants with the implanting physician prior to surgery.

Death (also called mortality) is rare during the initial defibrillator-implant surgery, but it is a risk of any procedure. A real-world look at defibrillator implantations estimates a 0.8 to 1.7 percent death rate associated with defibrillator implantation (Ezekowitz 2007). Death rates may be increased (2 percent) in the extreme elderly aged greater than eighty years due to increased age-related mortality in this group (Stevenson et al. 2012). A more important discussion is the effect of procedure-related complications and death. As we discussed earlier, there can be as high as a 4 to 8 percent risk of major complications with defibrillator implantation depending on the physician and hospital performing the surgery. A recent study (Lee 2010) shows that a patient having a major complication can have a 10 to 20 percent death rate. This means that one to two people out of ten who have a major complication could die within six weeks of the defibrillator-implant surgery.

Complications that usually occur more than one month after implant.

Lead malfunction/Failures: Twiddling was originally described in 1968 (Bayliss et al. 1968) and refers to patient manipulation of the device can or leads that may result in malfunction. It has a reported incidence of 0.07 percent (seven out of ten thousand) in a large series of patients (Fahraeus and Hoijer 2003); however, I have seen almost one per year since I have been in practice. Figure 20 depicts lead orientation before and after patient twiddling resulted in lead dislodgement.

Exit block: Sometimes leads that pace require more voltage than normal to adequately pace the heart. Transient disruptions to the pacing function can be caused by systemic disease states (like infection) and electrolyte abnormalities, drug effects, extreme hypothyroidism (low thyroid), and coronary-artery disease (cardiac ischemia). There is an expected rise in voltage requirements in the two- to six-week period after lead placement attributed to local inflammation or foreign-body reaction at the tip-tissue interface. The degree to which the capture threshold increases is markedly blunted with steroid-eluting leads, which have thus become generally preferred for their more favorable delivery characteristics, having overcome the problem of higher stimulation thresholds (Ellenbogen et al. 1999; Fortescue et al. 2005).

It is noteworthy that most current leads are active fixation (meaning the lead is actively fixed to the heart by a corkscrew-like helix at the tip). These active-fixation leads tend to have a slightly higher pacing requirement. Passive-fixation leads (see chapter 4) have capture thresholds relatively lower than standard active-fixation leads. The disadvantages to passive-fixation leads are an inability to perform atrial mapping, unreliable lateral-wall stability, and requirement for placement in the atrial appendage—which may be difficult in patients who have undergone bypass. A rise in capture threshold may occur beyond six weeks after implantation: the chronic phase of lead maturation. As the threshold steadily rises, it may exceed the maximum output of the pulse generator, and this is known as *exit block*. Exit block is recognized by high pacing thresholds without radiographic evidence of dislodgement (lead moves from its initial implant position). It may be related to inflammation or fibrosis at the site where it is attached to the inside of your heart (electrode-myocardium interface) and generally presents greater than four weeks after implantation (Hayes and Vliestra 1993). Some patients—particularly pediatric patients—are particularly prone to this phenomenon, and multiple lead revisions may be required for them.

Device/Lead advisories. See chapter 11.

Infection. Infection is estimated to occur in 1 to 2 percent of patients (one or two patients out of one hundred will get a device infection). Of these infections, up to 60 percent of patients present with localized infections involving their device pockets, whereas the remaining patients may present with endovascular (within the bloodstream) infections but no evidence of inflammation of their device pockets (Tarakji et al. 2010). Approximately 10 percent of patients may have intracardiac vegetations (collections of infected material) identified by transesophageal echocardiogram, though they can still undergo lead explantation safely (Grammes et al. 2010). The risk of defibrillator infection is higher than that of pacemakers. The presence of epicardial leads (placed on the outside of the heart during open-heart surgery) and postoperative complications at the generator pocket (e.g., pocket hematoma) are significant risk factors for early-onset device infection, whereas longer duration of hospitalization at the time of implantation and chronic obstructive pulmonary disease were associated with late-onset device infections (Williams and Stevenson 2012). In one of the largest studies of device infections (Johansen et al. 2011), repeated operative procedures after the first device implantation were associated with a substantial incremental risk of infection. Female gender, older age, and preoperative antibiotics given at the initial implant were associated with a lower risk of later infection. The pacing mode, indication for device, and complexity of the procedure were not independently associated with the risk of later infection. Sixty percent of infections have been found to occur within ninety days of implant (Nery et al. 2010), though a large number of infections occur during the late stage (greater than one year postimplant; Johansen et al. 2011). Generator changes and cardiac resynchronization therapy/dual-chamber devices have also been implicated as independent predictors of infection (Nery et al. 2010). In the first 1275 device implantations performed in our Heart Rhythm Center, we had only four devices (0.3 percent) develop infections within twelve months! Obviously, we do not want *any* devices to get infected, but this is a very low rate of device infection; we take extraordinary precautions to minimize the risk of device infections because treatment of device infections is very risky.

The generally accepted means of device infection treatment is removal of the generator and all implanted leads (Wilkoff 2007). In a large series of device extractions, including 1,838 leads (Grammes et al. 2010), postoperative thirty-day mortality was 10 percent, although no deaths were related directly to the extraction procedure. Another series of device extractions reported: a 0.5 percent rate of intraprocedural mortality, a 4.6 percent rate of in-hospital mortality, and a 2.6 percent rate of relapsing infections within one year of reimplantation (Tarakji et al. 2010). *Device infection is a very serious complication,* and any worrisome symptoms—such as fever, chills, redness, or drainage of the incision—should be reported to your doctor. I generally recommend that patients refrain from taking showers or tub baths within seven days of a device implantation, and I do not recommend any water, ointments, or salves near the incision during this time.

Pacemaker syndrome. This syndrome can occur with defibrillators, most commonly with single-chamber ventricular defibrillators (e.g., VVI or VVIR modes). Symptoms are due to loss of atrioventricular (AV) synchrony. The loss of AV synchrony means that the top chambers of your heart (the atria) may be pumping against contracting bottom chambers (the ventricles), which leads to uncomfortable symptoms. It must be noted that pacemaker syndrome can occur with any pacing mode if AV synchrony is lost. Symptoms include malaise, weakness, chest pain, cough, confusion, or syncope (fainting).

Venous thrombosis. Upper-extremity, deep-venous thrombosis (or stenosis) is uncommon in the general population without implantable devices, but venous stenosis (blockage) has been seen in up to 33 to 64 percent of patients after implantation of device leads (Oginosawa, Abe, and Nakashima 2002; DaCosta et al. 2002). Statistically significant factors that have been associated with an increased risk include: previous transvenous temporary leads (DaCosta et al. 2002), left-ventricular ejection fraction less than 40 percent (DaCosta et al. 2002), systemic infection (Bracke et al. 2003), absence of anticoagulation (blood thinners), use of hormone treatment, personal history of venous thrombosis, and presence of multiple leads (van Rooden et al. 2004). Symptoms may include shoulder or neck discomfort, ipsilateral (same side as defibrillator) arm swelling with cyanosis (bluish discoloration), dilated, collateral cutaneous veins around the shoulder, or jugular-vein distension (Rozmus et al. 2005). Venography (using IV contrast) is considered the gold standard for diagnosis, but compressive ultrasonography (noninvasive test using sonagraphy or ultrasound) is an effective and economical means of confirming the clinical diagnosis (Rozmus et al. 2005). Veins that develop blood clots (thrombosis) can develop blood-flow limiting blockages (called *stenosis*). If a stenosis is severe enough, the blood vessel can close and this is called an *occlusion*. Treatment may include: anticoagulation (warfarin and/or heparin), extraction of the old nonfunctioning lead to create a new venous channel, or venoplasty to reduce venous stenosis or allow the implantation of subsequent leads (Rozmus et al. 2005; Worley et al. 2011).

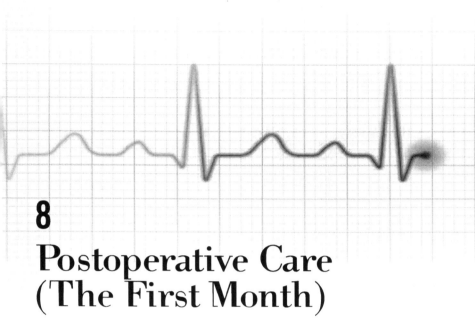

8

Postoperative Care (The First Month)

Each implanting physician and practice will have slightly different postoperative-care instructions, and it is important to check with your doctor regarding special instructions after defibrillator implantation. The limitations/restrictions I generally recommend to patients following defibrillator implantation are summarized in this chapter. But sometimes my postoperative care varies, depending on a particular patient's medical problems. You should confirm activity limitations/restrictions with your own doctor after the device implantation.

Care of the incision (showering/bathing). Proper healing of the incision is critical to avoid infections after the implantation. For this reason, I recommend no tub baths or showers for seven days after the implantation—the average duration of restriction ranges from two to fourteen days. The patient should not get water, soap, ointments, or salves on or near the incision during this time (unless instructed otherwise by the implanting physician). I often joke with my patients, "Stink it up! If you smell nice when you come back for the wound check, I know you cheated." This is an exaggeration, but proper postoperative wound care is critical for a successful defibrillator implantation; see chapter 7 for a discussion on the risks of device infections. Once the incision has healed during this initial period, the patient can begin showering, and any superficial bandages (e.g., Steri-Strips®) will begin to fall off on their own. I usually use three layers of absorbable sutures (stitches) to close the incision, and these will slowly get absorbed by the body during the normal healing process. Some doctors use staples to close the skin layer of a pacemaker incision; the patient will have to return to the doctor's office in one to two weeks to remove the staples. The same bathing instructions apply to patients with staples in place.

It is normal for the incision to be sore after device implantation. There will be mild tenderness at the incision site that should be improving on a daily basis. If the pain is getting worse or the incision gets redder or more swollen or feels hot, the patient should call the implanting physician. The vast majority of my patients require only non-narcotic pain relief (e.g., Advil® or Tylenol®)

after the implantation, but some patients may require a few days of narcotic pain relief after the implantation.

The incision itself may look slightly red for the first several days, but each day it should get less and less red. If there is any increasing redness, warmth, or swelling, the implanting physician should be notified. You may see some dried blood along the incision, and this can be normal; if bleeding persists or the incision continues to ooze or leak fluid, the implanting physician should be notified. Figure 19 depicts examples of both normal (figure 19A) and abnormal incisions and device pockets (figure 19C–F). You can typically see (and feel) the outline of the device (and sometimes the leads in thin patients) and mild soft-tissue swelling in a pocket that is healing normally. There should be no significant tension on the incision; the incision should not look like it is being "stretched" because of swelling underneath. A pocket hematoma is an abnormal collection of blood around the device, but underneath the incision, that looks like swelling. You can see exaggerated fullness around a device with a hematoma present (figure 19F); you will not see such fullness in a normally healing defibrillator site. Finally, some thin patients may only have a very thin layer of skin over the healed device site (Figure 19B), and you may even see the course of the defibrillator lead. As long as there is no abnormal redness or tenderness, this can be a normal finding. Again, any concern about the incision healing should be relayed to your doctor.

Symptoms that should be reported immediately to a physician:

- Fevers or chills

- Incisional redness, warmth, tenderness, or swelling

- Drainage or bleeding from the incision site

- Chest pain, shortness of breath, difficult breathing

- Hiccups or abnormal "twitching" of chest-wall or rib-cage muscles

- Swelling in arms, wrists, legs, or ankles

- Fainting (syncope), lightheadedness, or dizziness

- Palpitations or fast, racing heartbeat

- Severe weakness or fatigue

- Any dramatic change or development of symptoms immediately following an implant

Activity limitations. Patients should not raise the implant-side arm above shoulder height or behind their backs for four weeks after the implantation. In addition, I recommend that patients not lift more than five pounds (or a gallon of milk) during these four weeks. These restrictions give the defibrillator leads a chance to scar in place. It must be noted that it can take up to six weeks for the leads to become securely anchored in the pocket. In addition, it may take several months for the leads to become scarred in place in the heart. Any sudden trauma (such as a fall or car accident) within the first several months after implantation can cause defibrillator-lead dislodgement. Contact sports and vigorous activity should be avoided during the first four weeks. In fact, I generally recommend that contact sports (e.g., football and rugby) and vigorous activity that involves significant jarring (e.g., horseback riding or jackhammer use) be avoided in any patients who have a defibrillator. You should ask your doctor about participating in any activity that may involve excessive jarring or trauma.

Driving. I generally recommend that patients not drive until the first follow-up appointment: ten to fourteen days after implantation. This allows me to make sure the incision is healing properly and leads are functioning appropriately. Obviously, patients who experienced any alterations in consciousness (fainting) prior to receiving the defibrillator implantation should not drive until their physicians deem it safe to do so. Each state is different; Pennsylvania law, for example, suggests that patients may drive after six months if the reason for their fainting (syncope) can be fully explained and they have no further episodes of syncope during this time. It is recommended that the patient not drive for twelve months from the last episode of fainting if no cause is identified. Please check with your doctor before you resume driving.

The first follow-up appointment after the defibrillator implantation. The patient usually receives a card describing the maker of the device and leads; this is important information to know in case of an emergency. A follow-up visit is usually arranged for one to two weeks from the device implant. I have the patient return for a visit with our device clinic to assess the incision, check the device, and continue the defibrillator-education process. Some patients are required to follow up with separate doctors for the incision check (if a surgeon implanted the device) and device check (performed at the cardiologist's or primary-care provider's office). After this initial visit, the patient will be scheduled for an in-office device evaluation and ongoing education at three months post-implant. These evaluations may occur over the phone (transtelephonic monitoring), wirelessly (via cell phone service or Internet), or in person if the device cannot be remotely monitored. Each physician offers different follow-up options. Most of the new devices offer remote monitoring via a secure website. This allows patients to have their devices checked from home. Remote monitoring is especially convenient for patients whose mobility or transportation options are limited.

These visits/checks allow your doctor to make sure the device and leads are working appropriately and the battery is OK. Moreover, remote monitoring can allow your doctor to track your heart failure and detect arrhythmias, such as atrial fibrillation.

Lifestyle considerations. One major concern for many patients is that defibrillators will dramatically affect their lifestyles. Once temporary activity limitations are lifted (generally at four weeks), there are very few changes that need to be made. First, most home-electronic devices are safe for use around a defibrillator. Any properly grounded, handheld electronic device is safe as long as it is kept a safe distance from the defibrillator site—approximately six inches is a good rule of thumb. Microwave ovens are safe to use (and I jokingly tell patients, "As long as you don't climb inside!"). Induction ovens may emit noise that can interfere with a defibrillator, and you should stay several feet away from a working induction oven. Any device that has electrical output (arc welding is an example) could cause defibrillator malfunction. The most common malfunction is that the interfering device causes the pacemaker to "oversense" noise and fool the defibrillator into delivering a shock. It is also possible for defibrillators to not function as pacemakers during such noisy periods. I have seen this happen with transcutaneous electrical nerve stimulators (TENS units). Another malfunction I have seen involves improper household grounding. During flooding in our region, a defibrillator patient went into a flooded basement, and the device inappropriately recognized external noise (from a shorted furnace) as a life-threatening arrhythmia and delivered a shock while the patient was awake! Needless to say this is very dangerous *and* uncomfortable for the patient. Most home power tools are safe to use when kept at arm's length;

however, gas-powered tools (especially chain saws) may cause interference with defibrillators. Check with your doctor prior to using any gas-powered tools or other devices that may emit electrical noise.

I do not recommend that patients linger in or near the security exits of stores; there is a slim chance of electrical noise from these areas. There are several situations that can interfere with defibrillator operation, and table 4 lists many procedures that may interfere with your defibrillator. Arc welding produces large amounts of electrical noise, and you cannot expose a defibrillator to these fields. This electrical noise can cause your defibrillator to stop pacing and/or inappropriately shock you. If you think an electric field is affecting defibrillator function, you should move away from the source of the noise. Any powerful electrical or magnetic field can interfere with a defibrillator. Companies are developing MRI-approved defibrillators that may safely allow a patient to undergo an MRI scan. Interestingly, there are some centers that will allow patients with an existing defibrillator to undergo MRI scanning, but every center is different. Please check with your doctor about MRI scanning and your future need for MRI scans. Your doctor may consider an MRI-approved defibrillator system.

I advise patients to avoid any activity that involves rough physical contact. Strenuous activities such as basketball, football, tennis, or racquetball could cause jarring and damage to the defibrillator or leads. In addition, you would not want to use a rifle on the same side as your defibrillator. There have been studies that suggest that younger patients and females in general have a higher rate of lead malfunction that is likely due to more intense physical activity and/or body shape/size. Finally, if you are unsure whether an activity/environment is safe for a defibrillator, please check with your doctor.

Table 4. Procedures That May Interfere with Defibrillator Function. This table describes many procedures that defibrillator patients undergo. These are meant as general guidelines. Always discuss the safety of any procedure with your doctor if you have a defibrillator.

Safe	Low Risk	Medium/High Risk	Unsafe
Dental procedures	CAT Scans	Electrocautery	MRI
X-rays	Ventilators (Breathing machines)	Hearing aids with coil around neck	Diathermy (Tissue heating that may be used by chiropractor)
In-ear hearing aids	Ultrasound	Tissue ablation	Arc welding
Mammography	Electrolysis	Lithotripsy	
	Handheld electronics (see below)	Radiation therapy	
		TENS units	

Can handheld electronics interfere with your defibrillator? The short answer is yes. We used to worry about noise from patients who do arc welding (this is still a no-no for defibrillator patients) but now a much more common risk for device interference is handheld electronics. Any device that has a magnet (such as earbuds or iPads™) may interfere with device function if placed directly over the defibrillator. It is important for a defibrillator patient to not fall asleep with a handheld electronic device directly over the defibrillator. Generally, most handheld electronics are safe if held more than twelve inches from the device. *If you feel any odd symptoms while using a handheld electronic, immediately move away from the device. If you are unsure about the safety of any electronic device, check with your doctor.*

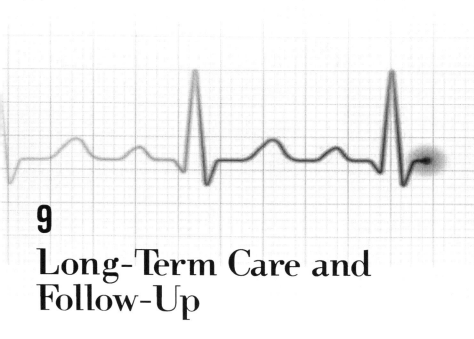

9
Long-Term Care and Follow-Up

Follow-up. As described in chapter 8, patients will have regularly scheduled defibrillator evaluations every three to twelve months. Regular follow-up is essential for defibrillator patients; this is so important that guidelines recommend a defibrillator *not* be placed in patients who cannot or will not be compliant with regular, postimplantation device care! Long-term, postimplant follow-up ensures optimal device performance, and allows us to follow devices under advisories, minimize complications, and permit appropriate patient tracking as well as detection of clinical problems in a timely manner. These evaluations may be performed in the office or performed remotely (from the patient's home). Defibrillator programming, lead function, and battery strength are routinely checked as well as any malfunction or manufacturer alert (see chapter 11 to learn about recalls/advisories). Many practices (including mine) schedule remote monitoring on a three-month basis to follow patients closely for possible lead malfunction, battery life, arrhythmias, and any other additional alerts the defibrillator has been programmed to monitor. Newer devices offer the ability for the defibrillator to track the patient's weight (requires a scale designed for that device), volume status (by measuring chest-wall impedance), and respiratory rate. These parameters can help your doctor monitor for heart failure.

Defibrillator function. During a routine defibrillator interrogation (remotely or in the office, see figure 11), your defibrillator function will be evaluated in a systematic way. First, the device-clinic staff will place a wand over the defibrillator site—some newer devices are fully wireless—and download a current status update for the defibrillator. This initial report will reveal any alerts/warnings that occurred since the last check as well as parameters that help us determine the remaining battery life and lead functions. The leads are evaluated based upon three main characteristics: 1) amplitude, 2) threshold, and 3) impedance.

> *Amplitude*: This refers to the voltage that your heart creates during a normal heartbeat. The size (or amplitude) of this voltage helps us determine how to program your device as well as how the lead is functioning. If the amplitude becomes too small, the defibrillator may not be able to detect your native

heartbeat. If the device cannot sense your native heartbeat (called *undersensing*), it may pace excessively or fail to deliver a lifesaving therapy for VT/VF.

Threshold: This refers to how much energy (voltage and current) is required to cause your heart to beat (we call this *capture*). The lower the threshold, the less energy required to pace your heart and the longer the battery life.

Impedance: This is a measure of the opposition in current that is present in the defibrillator lead. In other words, a normally functioning defibrillator lead has a certain range of normal impedance. An abnormal drop in this impedance may represent breakdown of the insulating material of the lead. An abnormal increase in impedance may represent a defect in the defibrillator's wires.

Patient monitoring features of defibrillators.

Arrhythmia burden: Most defibrillators have the ability to detect and record any occurrences of arrhythmias: such as atrial fibrillation or ventricular tachycardia. Often, the first time atrial fibrillation is detected is from the defibrillator's alerts.

Hemodynamic monitoring: Many defibrillators have the ability to monitor daily patient activity, volume status (via thoracic impedance), heart rates, and respiratory rates. The ability to track hemodynamic parameters like this can help us to make adjustments to medications.

Lead/Device advisories: Most defibrillators have alarms programmed that will alert us to possible lead or device problems: such as lead damage, battery/circuit failure, or software malfunctions. These alerts are reviewed during defibrillator checks.

Incision care. Generally, incisions have mostly healed four to six weeks after the defibrillator implantation, but it is important to routinely check your incision. Scarring can be minimized by applying sunscreen over the healed incision; check with your physician for when it is safe to apply sunscreen to your incision. Any cracking, oozing, bleeding, swelling, or redness should be reported immediately to your physician. Protect your incision and device pocket from any direct trauma or abrasion—from seatbelts in particular. Any device trauma should be reported to your physician, and device check should be performed remotely or in the office (to permit an examination of the incision and device pocket).

If your car's shoulder seatbelt crosses directly over where your device sits, it is worthwhile to use a sheepskin seatbelt cover to prevent *pocket erosion*. Pocket erosion is caused by thinning of the skin and tissue overlying the pacemaker (figure 19B) that can ultimately lead to skin breakdown (figure 19D); it exposes the defibrillator and leads to bacteria from the skin's surface. Pocket erosions (figure 19E) generally mandate complete device (and lead) removal (called *extraction*). Defibrillator extractions can be very dangerous and risky to the patient.

Finally, the patient should never manipulate (called *twiddling*) the device or leads. Patients who twiddle the defibrillator (e.g., roll it over or slide it side to side in the pocket) can damage the leads and/or defibrillator. Figure 20 shows retracted right- and left-ventricular leads tangled in the pocket superior to a defibrillator that has been rotated by twiddling. Leads may become dislodged and malfunction—requiring reoperation.

Battery/Lead life. The battery of a defibrillator is sealed within the metal can that includes the defibrillator circuitry (see figure 7). When the battery is depleted, the entire defibrillator is replaced; the existing leads are reused if they are working fine with no obvious damage. This involves opening the prior incision, disconnecting the existing leads, and attaching a new defibrillator to these leads. This procedure can usually be done as an outpatient, with the patient returning home later in the day. I generally have patients continue all their medications (including anticoagulation with warfarin), but check with your own physician regarding your medication regimen.

Defibrillator batteries generally last from three to eight years—depending on how much pacing or how many defibrillator shocks the patient requires. I have had defibrillators last ten to fifteen years if the patient is rarely being paced and has not had any shocks. Unless there is an advisory, alert, or recall (discussed in chapter 11), defibrillator batteries slowly run out, and depletion can be detected during routine device checks. Once the defibrillator reaches the Elective Replacement Indicator (ERI), it will generally continue to function for three months— allowing time to schedule the generator-replacement procedure.

Defibrillator leads can have a variable life-span. Often, the leads outlast the defibrillator itself and are reused with the new defibrillator during a defibrillator generator replacement. Prior to any defibrillator replacement, the leads are reevaluated to be sure they function properly and to determine whether there are any recalls/advisories/alerts as to possible malfunction. It must be noted that there can be a fourfold increase in lead malfunction after a generator change due to the manipulation of leads required during the procedure.

Traveling. It is OK to travel by air and go through security checkpoints with a defibrillator, but I recommend that patients do not walk through the metal detector. I recommend that they show their defibrillator ID cards to security and have security do "wand checks" for metal objects (with care not to place the metal-detection wand directly over the device). Routine defibrillator follow-up visits are very important, so if you plan to be away from home for several weeks to months, ask your physician to help you find a physician at your travel destination who will be available for unexpected health issues. Most defibrillator companies have an international presence for emergency-device checks, but discuss international travel plans with your doctor, and find out about any heart centers that are near your destination.

Can a defibrillator worsen heart failure? Yes, but it is not common. Usually a person's heart has electrical activation from top to bottom. When a person is dependent on the pacing features of a defibrillator, the very tip of the bottom-right chamber (right ventricle) is paced first; this causes the heart muscle to be activated in an unnatural sequence (called *dyssynchrony*). There have been studies that confirm RV pacing can cause mild heart failure as seen by an approximate 11 percent drop in ejection fraction (Fung et al. 2007). Patients at risk of heart failure because of defibrillator pacing (i.e., they have heart block or slow heart rates) may benefit from a resynchronization defibrillator by having an additional lead placed in the left ventricle (biventricular pacing). This is called a *biventricular defibrillator* and consists of three leads: leads in the right atrium, right ventricle, and the extra lead in the left ventricle (placed via the coronary sinus). This special type of defibrillator has been demonstrated to treat and prevent progression of heart failure in many patients (Moss et al. 2009; Yu et al. 2009; Curtis et al. 2013). You should talk to your doctor to see if this is an appropriate option for you. Not all patients need this special type of defibrillator. There are some other rare causes of heart failure from defibrillators, and you can ask your doctor if you are at risk for this.

What should I do if the defibrillator shocks me (or my loved one)?

Approximately 20 to 30 percent of defibrillator patients will receive therapies (either shocks or antitachycardia pacing) within two years of device implantation (Goldenberg et al. 2006). The occurrence of shocks may be higher or lower depending on the reason the defibrillator was implanted. These are the general instructions patients can be given as a "shock plan":

1. If you receive a shock and have symptoms after the shock, go to the emergency room immediately. Call 911; do not drive yourself.

2. If you have multiple shocks within a short period of time (within the hour), go to the emergency room immediately. Call 911; do not drive yourself.

3. If you have a shock with no symptoms or felt symptoms but no shock, call the device clinic, and your doctor will try to schedule an ICD check within the next twenty-four hours.

4. If you have a shock with no symptoms after hours or on the weekend, call the device-clinic answering service (most often your care providers' general answering service). The answering service will take your message and direct it to

the care provider on call. The care provider will call you with instructions for follow-up. He/she may ask that you go to the hospital emergency room. The defibrillator company representative may be called to check your device in order to provide more information to the physician. You should call the device clinic on the next business day for continuity of your defibrillator care.

Symptoms to worry about may include lightheadedness, dizziness, feeling faint, chest pain, or shortness of breath, feeling symptoms similar to those experienced before the defibrillator was implanted, or not feeling well after the shock.

Inappropriate therapies or shocks happen when the defibrillator is fooled into thinking a patient is having a life-threatening arrhythmia. Approximately 10 to 15 percent of defibrillator patients may receive a therapy (shock or antitachycardia pacing) for a generally nonfatal arrhythmia (Goldenberg et al. 2006). There are three common situations that may lead to a defibrillator mistakenly shocking a patient.

1. *Atrial fibrillation or other arrhythmias from the top chamber (the atria) causing inappropriate therapies*: If a patient has atrial fibrillation causing a very fast heart rate (like during a period of infection), the defibrillator activates special types of discriminating tools (built into the device cir-

cuitry) that try to decide if this is a potentially fatal arrhythmia. If the heart rate continues to be very fast (often greater than 200 bpm), the device ultimately makes the decision to err on the cautious side and deliver a shock. Not only can these shocks terminate the fatal arrhythmias (VT/VF), but they may well terminate the atrial fibrillation.

2. *Noise or artifact causing inappropriate therapies*: Noise external to the patient (such as interfering electrical signals from arc welding) or lead malfunctions (such as breaks in the lead wires) can simulate very fast heart rates. If the noise is sustained for several seconds, the device may be fooled into delivering a therapy.

3. *Exercise causing inappropriate therapies:* Soon after finishing my electrophysiology training and starting practice, I had a young patient get inappropriately shocked by his defibrillator while having sex! The patient was able to generate a very fast (though not dangerous) heart rhythm called *sinus tachycardia*. Sinus tachycardia is the rhythm that occurs during exercise. Understandably, this patient was very upset, and I reprogrammed his device to prevent this from recurring. To this day, I continue to use a high heart-rate cutoff (often based upon the patient's age) to minimize the risk of this happening again. There are other, less common causes of inappropriate therapies, and

your doctor can discuss these should they occur with your defibrillator.

Long-term psychosocial effects of defibrillators. Like any other serious medical condition or procedure, patients undergoing defibrillator implantation can develop emotional problems. See chapter 10 for discussion of possible psychosocial issues after defibrillator implantation.

Do defibrillators keep extremely elderly patients alive and prevent natural death? This will not occur when a patient and family's wishes are relayed to the patient's care providers. When a defibrillator patient becomes terminally ill, it is generally not the patient's (or family's) wish to prevent sudden death, which can often be a painless death. In this situation, we commonly deactivate the features of the defibrillator that prevent sudden cardiac death. It is very important to discuss deactivating the defibrillator when a patient enters hospice care. Hospice care provides care and support of a patient (both physically and emotionally) to enable comfort and dignity at the end of life.

The pacing function of defibrillators generally does not keep terminally ill patients alive. Most events that cause death at end of life are due to issues like overwhelming infection (sepsis), bleeding, cancer, strokes, or major organ failure (kidney or liver). During these types of catastrophic events, the heart is too sick to be paced by the defibrillator. The current ACC/AHA/HRS Guidelines on Device Therapy state: "Clinicians should encourage patients undergoing device implantation to complete advanced directives and specifically address the matter of device management and deactivation if the patient is terminally ill" (Epstein et al. 2008).

In cases where the patient, family, and/or clinician feel that the defibrillators are not providing the appropriate therapy/care (e.g., for patients with severe, debilitating dementias), deactivation of devices is an option. It must be noted that many patients are not dependent upon the pacing features of a defibrillator, and it is rare that deactivation results in immediate patient death. Often, when death is imminent, a patient's heart is racing and not relying on the pacemaker function. Finally, it is a patient's—or a patient's medical-decision-maker's—right to request the withdrawal of defibrillator support. Withdrawal of lifesaving defibrillator support with the informed consent of the patient is not considered euthanasia or physician-assisted suicide—though some doctors may be conscientious objectors (Epstein et al. 2008).

10
Psychosocial Impact of Defibrillators

In chapter 3 we talked about the reasons a defibrillator may be a lifesaving therapy. But a defibrillator could cause or worsen emotional distress.

Adjustment to life after defibrillator implantation. One of the most important aspects of a patient's life after defibrillator implantation is *acceptance* of the device. One can minimize this by saying "The device is implanted, and you have to get used to it!" Unfortunately, it is not this simple. Burns et al. (2005) define patient acceptance of a defibrillator as:

> "The psychological accommodation and understanding of the advantages and disadvantages of the device, the recommendation of the device to others,

and the derivation of benefit in terms of biomedical, psychological, and social functioning. Patient acceptance is theorized to be a device-specific component of the construct of quality of life."

This can be simplified to mean that patients have accepted their devices when they understand that the lifesaving benefits of the devices outweigh their risks and that quality of life is not negatively impacted by the devices. Not only can emotional stress cause cardiac events, but there is some evidence that certain personality traits can affect the long-term prognosis of defibrillator patients. Warning signs of patients who may have difficulty adjusting to their defibrillators (and possibly have more heart-rhythm abnormalities) include patients with high levels of preimplantation device-related concerns as well as individuals that experience excessive worrying, depression, negativity, and anxiety (Pedersen et al. 2010).

Quality of life in defibrillator patients. Quality of life refers to the general well-being of a patient. Most defibrillator trials evaluated the lifesaving effects of defibrillators but did not particularly study the effects of defibrillators on a patient's general well-being. Defibrillator patients have been found to have similar quality-of-life ratings as heart patients without defibrillators (Sears and Conti 2002; Groeneveld et al. 2007; Pedersen et al. 2009). Furthermore, the reason for defibrillator implantation (for example, a person with a history of sudden-death events versus a person with no such history) does not appear to affect patients' quality-of-life ratings. Patients planning to undergo defibrillator implantation should expect minimal negative impact of the defibrillator on their physical and emotional well-being (Groeneveld et al. 2007). It is important to note that patients may have anxiety about driving or lifting children (or heavy objects), and concerns about sexual activity (Groeneveld et al. 2007). It is important to discuss these concerns with your doctor. A majority of patients are able to return to work after defibrillator implantation (if they want to; Sears and Conti 2002). Anxiety can occur after defibrillator implantation, and it is often due to the fear of prior shocks or the chance of a shock in the future.

Factors that may place patients at risk of significant psychosocial impact after defibrillator implant (Sears and Conti 2002):

- Female gender

- Age under fifty years

- History of a high rate of defibrillator shocks

- Poor knowledge of one's own cardiac condition or defibrillator

- History of psychological issues

- Poor social support (i.e., a lack of close family or friends)

- Other significant medical problems

How does defibrillator implantation affect your life partner? Not only can recipients of defibrillators experience depression or anxiety, but their life partners (or extended family) may also experience psychological issues surrounding defibrillator implantation. The majority of studies report that partner stress levels decrease in the first year after defibrillator implantation. Interestingly, defibrillator shocks do not appear to influence partners' quality of life, but the reason for defibrillator implantation and associated medical problems does seem to play more of a role in partner stress levels (van den Broek, Habibovic, and Pedersen 2010).

How do defibrillator shocks affect the patient? It is estimated that appropriate shocks (for possibly life-threatening arrhythmias) occur in 17 to 64 percent of defibrillator patients and inappropriate shocks (caused by nonlethal arrhythmias) occur in 10 to 24 percent of patients (Germano et al. 2006). Up to half of patients report at least some level of anxiety associated with the threat or actual experience of a shock (Lemon, Edelman, and Kirkness 2004). Indeed, patients who have received shocks may have slightly lower quality-of-life scores than patients who have not received shocks from their defibrillators (Sears and Conti 2002; Groeneveld et al. 2007).

Patients who experience anxiety about defibrillator shocks may demonstrate *avoidance behavior* (Lemon, Edelman, and Kirkness 2004) associated with:

1. *Places*: 15 to 20 percent of patients report avoiding specific places such as the gym, for fear of exercise-induced arrhythmias, or more public places, for fear of embarrassment.

2. *Associations*: the chance occurrence of a shock at, say, a picnic may cause patients to have an irrational fear of going to picnics so as to avoid a repeat event.

3. *Objects*: 27 percent of patients report avoiding certain objects they may falsely perceive as dangerous, such as mobile phones.

4. *Activities*: approximately 40 percent of patients may avoid activities such as exercise. Obviously, activities like scuba diving or horseback riding may not be recommended, but other forms of exercise are recommended for most heart failure patients.

If you and/or your loved one are avoiding situations that you used to enjoy, please discuss this with the implanting physician. Many defibrillator patients misinterpret perioperative defibrillator counseling and may be unnecessarily restricting their activities.

What are phantom shocks? Some patients experience the pain of a defibrillator shock when no shock was actually delivered by the device. This is called a *phantom shock*. As many as one in ten defibrillator patients have reported having phantom shocks (Kikkenborg Berg et al. 2013). Phantom shocks often occur during sleep (or at night), and so an explanation of these phantom shocks has been postulated as misinterpretation of sleep-onset muscle contractions that occur, for example, when you are nodding off to sleep and are suddenly startled awake. People with higher levels of depression and anxiety (Prudente et al. 2006) as well as recently implanted defibrillator patients (Kikkenborg Berg et al. 2013) may be more susceptible to phantom shocks. If you are diagnosed with having phantom shocks, it is important to realize that this is not a device malfunction or a danger, but you should discuss any concerns with your care provider.

Why is a shock plan important? The defibrillator provides constant monitoring for possibly fatal arrhythmias, and a shock likely indicates that the device is working properly. Although defibrillator patients generally have the same quality of life as patients without defibrillators, shocks have been linked to lower quality-of-life scores for some patients. Having a *shock plan* can help reduce anxiety and uncertainty about the defibrillator. The shock plan can help you and your care providers cope with a shock and give you an idea if you need to call your doctor or go to the emergency room.

A Typical Defibrillator Shock Plan

1. If you receive a shock and have symptoms after the shock, go to the emergency room immediately. Call 911; do not drive yourself.

2. If you have multiple shocks within a short period of time (i.e., within the hour), go to the emergency room immediately. Call 911; do not drive yourself.

3. If you have a shock with no symptoms or have felt symptoms but no shock, call the device clinic. Your doctor will try to schedule an ICD check within the next twenty-four hours.

4. If you have a shock with no symptoms after hours or on the weekend, call the device-clinic answering service (most often your care provider's general answering service). The answering service will take your message and direct it to the care provider on call. The care provider will call you with instructions for follow-up. He/she may ask that you go to the hospital emergency room. The defibrillator-company representative may be called to check your device in order to provide more information to the physician. You should call the device clinic on the next business day for continuity of your defibrillator care.

There are several things you can do to prepare for a defibrillator shock (Sears, Shea, and Conti 2005). First, *educate yourself* about everything about a defibrillator. The more you understand the reasons a defibrillator is implanted and how it can save your life, the more you can cope with a defibrillator shock. Second, make sure you carry complete record of *information about your health conditions*. You should always carry your defibrillator information card, a list of your medical conditions (including your most current ejection fraction), and a list of your current medications. *Rehearse an action plan* (or your shock plan) if your defibrillator delivers a shock. Talk to your doctor to make sure that you know what the doctor recommends for your shock plan. After you receive a shock, you should try *deep breathing to relax* in the time frame immediately following the shock. It is important to *discuss with your doctor* why you were shocked and if there are any medications or changes to device programming that can minimize the chance of getting another shock.

Defibrillators in children and young adults. Defibrillators can be used to prevent sudden death in children and young adults, but there are issues that may be particularly salient in young patients. It is important to convey to patients that defibrillators are lifesaving tools that can help them live long and healthy lives. The patient will benefit from a "strong community of family or friends" (Dimsdale et al. 2012). Family and friends should have a keen eye for any signs of anxiety or depression and not hesitate to seek out help if they are worried about the patient. As the children grow older, they will seek out more independence and need more information and control over their medical conditions. Family and friends should encourage the patient to participate in managing his or her own health (Dimsdale et al. 2012). Along the way, it is necessary to educate important adults in the child's life (for example, teachers, coaches, and family friends) about the defibrillator and the child's health condition.

Decisions about defibrillator implantation in children and young adults are particularly important not only from a quality-of-life standpoint but also due to lifelong issues with lead-related complications and for the sake of preserving vascular access for these patients. There is a higher incidence of appropriate and inappropriate therapies (shocks and pacing) in children and young adults (Korte et al. 2004). In the majority of cases this is due to nonfatal (nonventricular) arrhythmias and damage to the defibrillator leads. This may be due to the smaller size of the patients or the higher level of activity in a younger patient population.

Long-term acceptance of the defibrillator. The goal of your implanting physician and care-providing team is long-term acceptance of the device. Many defibrillator patients misinterpret exercise restriction, and education (like this book!) can help clear up misperceptions. (See table 4 in chapter 8 for activities that may negatively interact with your defibrillator) There may be local defibrillator support groups your implanting physician is aware of, and other patients' experiences with their defibrillator may offer helpful insight. A small percentage of patients may experience severe psychological issues (including avoidance behaviors), and counseling may be beneficial. It is important to alert your care provider for any psychological (and medical) issues that may arise after defibrillator implantation.

11
What are Device Recalls/ Advisories/Alerts?

Any time a defibrillator or lead may have a problem, it is placed under *advisory*. This term is used rather than *recall*, because the defibrillator or lead may have a small chance of failure. But for most patients, watchful waiting is the most appropriate option. Indeed, if a defibrillator or lead has to be replaced, the patient is subject to many of the same risks of the initial device implantation. A large, multicenter, Canadian observational study showed that the complication rate from device replacement for an advisory indication was an astounding 9.1 percent (Gould 2008). Of these, 5.9 percent required reoperation, and there were two deaths. Naturally, the risk of an adverse outcome during replacement must be balanced by the risk of death due to device malfunction. Pacemakers and defibrillators have saved thousands of lives, but, as is true of all devices, malfunctions will continue to occur.

In response to a marked increase in device advisories in 2005—and to balance alarmism with the continued protection of patients in high-risk situations—the Heart Rhythm Society (HRS) published guidelines in 2006 to aid physicians (Carlson and Wilkoff 2006). Arguably the most important outcome was a call for greater transparency of problems that occur with defibrillators that are currently in use and the reporting of failures, in recognition of the fact that physicians and patients need timely and accurate information regarding device performance. Device performance depends not only on the characteristics of the device but on the skill of the implanting physician and caregivers following the device (Carlson and Wilkoff 2006). Using data compiled from 1990–2002, FDA annual reports showed that confirmed device malfunctions leading to device explantation were about 0.1–0.9 percent for pacemakers (Carlson and Wilkoff 2006). There is a higher rate of advisories for defibrillators. Although failure rates are low, there is a negative psychological impact on patients who have a device that is under advisory.

To assist in communication from industry to physicians and patients, it was proposed that terminology be standardized. The term *recall* was changed to *Class I Advisory*, which is just short of a recommendation for device replacement because of a reasonable probability that malfunction could result in death or significant harm. *Class II* and *Class III* recalls are subsequently referred to as advisory notices (non–life-threatening malfunctions) and safety alerts (potential malfunctions). This information is disseminated from industry via standardized letters to physicians and patients; these letters are also available on the defibrillator manufacturer's website. Prior experience tells us the advisory information should be disseminated to physicians just before patients. Advisories should include general information about the malfunction and potential clinical implications, but they should acknowledge that treatment decisions should ultimately be determined by patients in consultations with physicians.

The situations where device replacement is recommended are (1) when the mechanism of malfunction is known and is likely to be recurrent or lead to patient death, (2) the patient is pacemaker-dependent, (3) the device was placed for a secondary prevention indication or has received appropriate therapy, or (4) the device is approaching EOL. Conservative management (enhanced noninvasive and remote monitoring) should be considered when (1) The rate of malfunction is very low in non-pacemaker-dependent patients, (2) the patient has significant comorbidities or high operative risk even when the risk of device malfunction is substantial, or (3) remote monitoring and software reprogramming can minimize risk (i.e., nonphysiologic noise).

If you are concerned about a potential advisory for your defibrillator (or leads), contact your doctor. Please note that doctors including myself often "mix and match" leads and defibrillators, and so your defibrillator may not be from the same manufacturer as the leads. If you hear about a company undergoing an advisory, it is important to be sure that it pertains to your particular defibrillator or lead.

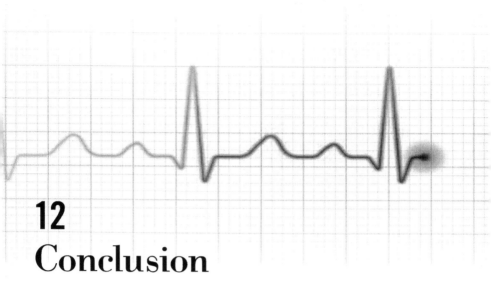

12
Conclusion

Defibrillators have saved countless lives and, as the population ages, more and more people will be living with advanced heart disease and needing defibrillators. Hopefully this comprehensive guide will provide patients and their families a full explanation of the "what, why, and how" of defibrillator implantation.

This book provides an in-depth study of defibrillators from initial patient evaluation through device implantation and the issues that may arise during long-term follow-up. I welcome the incorporation of this book into a typical plan of care for defibrillator patients beginning with initial discussions in the primary-care provider's office to serving as a long-term reference for patients who have received defibrillators. Indeed, I have found it a very useful complement to the informed-consent process of my patients during the consideration of defibrillator therapy.

Resources

Heart.org: This is the website for the American Heart Association. You will find exhaustive resources for physicians and patients about cardiovascular disease and stroke. The organization Fellows of the American Heart Association (denoted by FAHA after a doctor's name) recognizes a particular physician's scientific and professional accomplishments, volunteer leadership, and service dedicated to cardiovascular medicine.

Cardiosmart.org: This is the website for the American College of Cardiology. There is extensive information about cardiology for the patient and provider. Fellows of the American College of Cardiology (denoted by FACC after their names) are selected based on their outstanding credentials, achievements, and community contributions to promote excellence in cardiovascular care.

Hrsonline.org: The Heart Rhythm Society (HRS) is a leading resource on cardiac pacing, defibrillators, and electrophysiology. This specialty organization represents medical, allied health, and science professionals, from more than seventy countries, who specialize in heart-rhythm disorders. HRS delivers programs and services to its membership. Fellows of the Heart Rhythm Society (denoted by FHRS after their names) have advanced training, certifications, and demonstrated commitment to the research and treatment of heart-rhythm disorders.

Heart-rhythm-center.com: This is my discussion forum for biotechnology, pacemakers, defibrillators, and electrophysiology studies—including ablation. Patients and physicians can learn about and comment on a host of heart-rhythm-related topics.

Defibrillator-manufacturer websites: The following is a list of the most commonly implanted defibrillators and their websites. They often have patient and physician educational resources that are very informative:

1. Biotronik: www.biotronik.com

2. Boston Scientific Corporation: www.bostonscientific.com

3. Medtronic, Inc.: www.medtronic.com

4. Soren Group USA, Inc.: www.soren.com

5. St. Jude Medical, Inc.: www.sjm.com

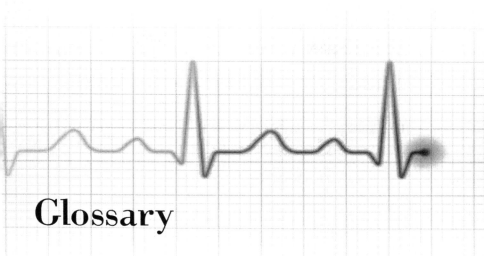

Glossary

<u>Ablation</u>: Catheter-based electrical heating of tissue that is used to treat arrhythmias in the electrophysiology laboratory.

<u>Advisory</u>: A warning issued to alert patients and care providers that a defibrillator or leads may be at risk for malfunction.

<u>Amplitude</u>: The level of voltage the heart generates or that a defibrillator lead delivers to the heart for pacing.

<u>Anaphylaxis</u>: Severe allergic reaction.

<u>Anticoagulation</u>: Thinning of the blood of a patient who may be on aspirin, warfarin, or heparin-based products.

<u>Antitachycardia pacing (ATP)</u>: Rapid pacing delivered by the defibrillator to painlessly terminate an arrhythmia.

<u>Aorta</u>: The large vessel leaving the heart that carries blood to the rest of the body.

<u>Aortic valve</u>: The valve that blood crosses when it is pumped out of the heart into the aorta.

<u>Arrhythmia</u>: Abnormal heart rhythm that may be too slow or too fast.

<u>Arrhythmogenic</u>: Characteristic of a medication, condition, or situation that can cause an abnormal heart rhythm.

<u>Asymptomatic</u>: Displaying a lack of symptoms.

<u>Atelectasis</u>: Minor collapse of lung airways that is common after surgeries and may cause fever or difficulty breathing.

<u>Atrioventricular (AV) block</u>: Electrical-conduction block between the top heart chambers (atrium) and the bottom heart chambers (ventricles). Pacing features of the defibrillator may be necessary when you have AV block.

<u>Atrioventricular (AV) node</u>: Specialized region of tissue that conducts electrical impulses from the top heart chambers (atrium) to the bottom heart chambers (ventricles).

Atrium: Either of the top chambers of the heart that pumps the blood to the ventricles (plural, atria).

Axillary vein: The main vein that drains the arm; when the axillary vein enters the rib cage, it forms the subclavian vein.

Basilic vein: This vein drains blood from the arm and joins with the cephalic vein to form the axillary vein.

Bifascicular block: Electrical-system block below the atrioventricular node in the right and left bundle branches.

Biventricular: Refers to both the left and right ventricles and is generally used to describe a defibrillator that resynchronizes the left and right ventricles in patients with or at risk for heart failure.

Bradycardia: An abnormally slow heart rate less than sixty beats per minute.

Brugada syndrome: A heart-rhythm disorder associated with electrocardiogram abnormalities that can cause sudden death.

Bundle branch: The left and right bundle branches are the major branches of the conduction system that provide electrical activation for the left and right ventricles;

the left bundle branch has two major subdivisions called the left-anterior and left-posterior fascicles.

Capture: Term describing when an electrical pacing signal (voltage and current) causes atrial or ventricular tissue to contract (depolarize).

Cardiac-resynchronization therapy (CRT): A technique that uses an extra lead in the left ventricle so that the right and left ventricles pump at the same time.

Cardioinhibitory response: A decrease in heart rate and blood pumping that can cause a loss of consciousness.

Cardiologist: Internal medicine doctor whose training involves four years of undergraduate college, four years of medical school, three years of internal medicine residency, and three years of cardiology fellowship.

Cardiomyopathy: A disease process that can cause a loss of heart-muscle pumping ability and lead to heart failure.

Cardioversion: A procedure using electricity or medicines to convert an abnormally fast heart rhythm to a normal rhythm.

Catecholaminergic polymorphic ventricular tachycardia: A rare condition that may cause sudden death during stress or physical exertion.

Catheter: Small tube that can be inserted in the heart via a peripheral blood vessel in the arm or leg.

Catheterization: The process by which catheters are placed into the heart's chambers or coronary arteries.

Cephalic vein: A large vein that is often seen in the upper arm over the bicep muscle and joins with the basilica vein to form the axillary vein; this vein runs in the groove between the shoulder and chest muscles (called the deltopectoral groove).

Chronotropic incompetence: An inability to increase heart rate during exercise or exertion.

Clavicle: The medical name for the collarbone; defibrillators are generally implanted two finger breadths below the clavicle.

Complete heart block: A complete lack of electrical communication between the atrium and ventricles that often requires pacing when it is irreversible.

Congenital: Any abnormal heart condition a person is born with.

Congestive heart failure: The heart's inability to pump enough blood to the rest of the body.

<u>Contraindication</u>: Medical reason that prevents a patient from having defibrillator implantation.

<u>Contrast</u>: Clear liquid that is used to highlight blood vessels and heart structure during defibrillator implantation.

<u>Contrast-induced nephropathy (CIN)</u>: Kidney damage that is caused by intravenous dye (called contrast) given during device implantation.

<u>Coronary artery</u>: Blood vessel that runs on the outside of the heart (epicardium) and provides oxygenated blood to the heart muscle; the left main coronary artery branches into the left-anterior descending and left circumflex: these generally supply blood to the left side of the heart (left atrium and ventricle); the right coronary artery generally supplies blood to the right side of the heart (right atrium and ventricle).

<u>Coronary sinus</u>: This is the major vein that drains blood from the heart muscle and directs it back toward the right atrium so blood can be reoxygenated in the lungs; the coronary sinus allows placement of pacemaker leads that are used to pace the left ventricle to enable resynchronization therapy.

<u>Creatinine</u>: A blood laboratory that indicates kidney function.

Current: Flow of electric charge through defibrillator leads.

Defibrillator: Device that is used to terminate life-threatening arrhythmias. A defibrillator can be fully implantable or applied externally by paramedics.

Diaphragm: Muscle responsible for causing the lungs to expand during breathing; the phrenic nerve can be inadvertently paced causing a "hiccup" sensation (called diaphragmatic stimulation).

Diastolic: Refers to the time of minimum blood pressure during relaxation of the heart between beats. Diastolic heart failure is when your heart does not relax effectively between heart beats.

Dislodgement: Term describing when a lead moves out of position after a defibrillator implantation, which may cause the lead to malfunction.

Dissection: Tear in a blood vessel that may require treatment.

Dyssynchrony: Failure of the right and left ventricles of the heart to contract at the same time; often present in heart-failure patients.

Echocardiogram: Special type of ultrasound (or sono-gram) that uses sound waves to assess the structure and function of the heart.

Edema: Swelling from excess fluid in your body's tissues. Edema may be found in your lungs, abdomen, hands or legs.

Effusion: Collection of blood or fluid around the heart or lungs.

Ejection fraction (EF): Amount of blood that is pumped by the heart during a normal heartbeat; a normal EF is between 55 and 70 percent.

Elective replacement indicator (ERI): Alert on a defibrilla-tor that signals it is necessary for the defibrillator genera-tor to be replaced; generally, a defibrillator can function several weeks to months once it reaches ERI.

Electrocardiogram (ECG): Apparatus that records the electrical activity of the heart, via electrodes that are placed on a patient's chest; the ECG is an important tool that cardiologists use to evaluate for disease.

Electrolyte: These are elements/minerals that are found in the blood and are important for normal heart func-tion; they can cause heart-rhythm abnormalities and are measured as part of routine laboratories in preparation for defibrillator implantation.

Electrophysiologist: Subspecialized cardiologist who has extra training and expertise to perform heart-rhythm evaluations and electrophysiology-device implants, such as pacemakers and defibrillators.

Electrophysiology: Study of heart rhythm disorders.

Electrophysiology study: Term describing a procedure in which a specialized cardiologist (cardiac electrophysiologist) places catheters inside the heart to record and assess the heart's electrical function.

End of life (EOL): Alert on a defibrillator that signifies that the battery is very close to empty; at EOL, the defibrillator can behave erratically and even fail.

Endocardium: The inside lining of the heart muscle that is in direct contact with the blood.

Epicardium: Outside lining of the heart that is in contact with the pericardium; coronary arteries are found here.

Erosion: Thinning of the skin over a defibrillator that can lead to infection.

Fascicle: Branches of the heart's conduction system that are called the left-anterior and posterior fascicles.

Fibrillation: Very fast beating of the heart that can be seen in the atrium (not generally fatal) or ventricle (often fatal).

Fistula: Abnormal connection between arteries and veins that can be caused by vascular access during heart procedures.

Fixation: Term describing how leads are attached to the heart during defibrillator implantation; active fixation involves a small helix that is screwed into the heart; passive fixation involves small, soft fingers that are wedged into the lining of the heart to stay attached (like the barbs of a fishhook).

Fluoroscopy: Special type of imaging that allows the doctor to perform x-rays while the patient or the heart is moving. Fluoroscopy is used during defibrillator implantation to place the leads into the heart.

Header: Block at the top of a defibrillator where the leads are connected.

Heart attack: Sudden blockage of a coronary artery, often referred to as an MI or myocardial infarction by care providers.

Hematoma: Abnormal collection of blood that can cause swelling of a defibrillator pocket under the skin.

Hemodynamics: Study of blood flow and the body's circulation; some pacemakers have features that can detect hemodynamic indicators such as fluid retention, activity, and respiratory motion.

Hemothorax: Abnormal collection of blood around the lungs in the chest that can result from a defibrillator implantation; it can be detected by a chest x-ray.

High-frequency jet ventilation: A special form of ventilation that is used to minimize respiratory motion during a surgical procedure.

His purkinje: Fibers of the conduction system in the bottom heart chambers (ventricles).

Hydration: Overall water content of a patient and/or the process of replacing or adding to the water content of a patient.

Hypertension: Elevated blood pressure.

Hyperthyroid: Abnormally elevated thyroid function.

Hypertrophic cardiomyopathy: Type of heart disease that causes a much thickened heart muscle and can cause sudden death (particularly in young athletes).

Hypotension: Low blood pressure.

Hypothyroid: Abnormally decreased thyroid function.

Impedance: Measure of the opposition in current that is present in the defibrillator lead.

Indication: Medical reason for a defibrillator implantation.

Infarction: Dead heart-muscle cells caused by a heart attack; another name for a heart attack is myocardial infarction.

Inappropriate shock or therapy: Occurrence of unnecessary (and potentially harmful) shocks or pacing when the defibrillator erroneously senses (is "fooled into" thinking) that a patient is having a life-threatening arrhythmia.

Interrogation: Process of checking the function of an implanted defibrillator; it can be done at the bedside, in the office, or remotely while the patient is at home.

Ischemic cardiomyopathy: Heart failure caused by blocked coronary arteries.

Long-QT syndrome: Disease of heart-muscle cells that leads to electrocardiogram abnormalities and is a cause of sudden, unexpected death.

Mitral valve: One-way valve that blood crosses when traveling from the left atrium to left ventricle.

Mixed cardiomyopathy: Heart failure that has more than one cause, such as heart failure due to a combination of coronary-artery blockages and a leaking valve.

Morbidity: Risk of complications, injuries, or symptoms from a device implantation.

Mortality: Risk of death from a device implantation.

Myocardium: Heart muscle. Myocardial cells make up the myocardium.

Myopotential: Electrical potential that is created by muscle outside the heart—such as the diaphragm—that can be sensed by a defibrillator and cause an inappropriate shock or pause in pacing.

Nephropathy: Damage to the kidneys.

Nonischemic cardiomyopathy: Heart failure in a patient with no significant coronary-artery blockages.

Occlusion: Stoppage of blood flow through a blood vessel. If a *stenosis* is severe enough, the blood vessel can close off and result in occlusion.

Oversensing: Abnormal detection of signals by a defibrillator that can cause malfunction.

P wave: Component of the electrocardiogram that corresponds to the activation and contraction of the top heart chambers (right and left atria).

<u>Pacemaker</u>: Device that is used to maintain a normal heart rate.

<u>Perforation</u>: Hole in one of the heart's chambers, arteries, or veins.

<u>Pericardiocentesis</u>: Process of removing an abnormal collection of blood (pericardial effusion) surrounding the heart.

<u>Pericardium</u>: Thin sac that lines the outside of the heart; blood collecting between the outside of the heart and this lining is called a pericardial effusion.

<u>Phantom shock</u>: Pain of a defibrillator shock experienced by the patient when no shock was actually delivered by the device.

<u>Phlebitis</u>: Inflammation or irritation of a blood vessel.

<u>Phrenic nerve</u>: Nerve that controls the diaphragm.

<u>Pleura</u>: Thin linings that surround the lungs and other organs inside the chest.

<u>Pneumothorax</u>: Abnormal collection of air outside the lungs that can be seen after a pacemaker implantation.

<u>Primary prevention</u>: Prevention of the first occurrence of a fatal arrhythmia in a patient with risk factors.

Programmer: Desktop computer that is used to interrogate a defibrillator to check function and program pacemaker features.

Prophylaxis: Medication used to prevent a reaction or infection.

Pulmonary valve: One-way valve that blood crosses when traveling from the right ventricle to the lungs.

Pulse width: Duration of a signal, in milliseconds, that is used to pace the heart.

QRS complex: Component of the electrocardiogram that corresponds to the activation and contraction of the bottom heart chambers (right and left ventricles).

Resynchronization: Pacing feature that restores the pumping action of the heart so the right and left ventricles pump at the same time.

Secondary prevention: Prevention of another occurrence of a fatal arrhythmia in a patient who has had an initial event.

Shock plan: Action plan for what to do when upon receiving a shock from a defibrillator.

Shocks: Term describing the defibrillator's method to terminate arrhythmias by delivering bursts of high voltages to "reset" the heart and stop the harmful arrhythmias. They may be painful if the patient is conscious during shocks.

Short-QT syndrome: Heart-rhythm disorder associated with electrocardiogram abnormalities that can cause sudden death.

Sinoatrial (SA) node: Natural pacemaker of the heart located in the right atrium.

Sleep apnea: Sleep disorder that causes pauses or abnormally slow breathing during sleep.

Stenosis: Blockage in a vein or artery. Device leads can cause the veins they are placed in to become stenosed.

Stethoscope: Tool used by care providers to listen to the heart.

Stroke: Stoppage of blood flow to a part of the brain; strokes are also called transient ischemic attacks (TIA) or "brain attacks."

Subclavian vein: The vein located under the collarbone that carries blood to the heart; it is used to implant defibrillator leads.

Subcutaneous defibrillator: Special type of defibrillator that does not involve leads placed through the chest wall into the venous system. This is a type of defibrillator that does not offer routine pacing ability.

Sudden cardiac death: An unexpected death due to heart issues that occurs within one hour of symptom onset. A person can survive a sudden cardiac death if resuscitation with a defibrillator is performed quickly.

Supraventricular: Characteristic of electrical activation starting in the upper chambers of the heart (the right and left atria).

Synchrony: Simultaneous pumping of the right and left ventricles.

Syncope: Loss of consciousness; fainting.

Systolic: Refers to the time of maximum blood pressure during contraction of the heart. Systolic heart failure is when your heart cannot contract strongly enough.

T wave: Component of the electrocardiogram that corresponds to the relaxation and resetting of the bottom heart chambers (right and left ventricles).

Tachycardia: Abnormally fast heart rate above one hundred beats per minute.

Tachycardia-induced cardiomyopathy: Heart failure caused by an arrhythmia (such as atrial fibrillation) that causes the heart to beat very fast for sustained periods of time.

Tamponade: Dangerous pressure buildup outside the heart when blood collects between the outside of the heart (epicardium) and the sac that contains the heart (pericardium).

Therapies: Features that defibrillators use to terminate ventricular arrhythmias. Therapies include antitachycardia pacing and shocks.

Threshold: Energy (voltage and current) required to cause the heart to beat (this is called capture).

Thrombosis: Blood clot.

Tilt-Table Test: Method to evaluate causes for syncope that involves placing a patient on a table that tilts up to a steep angle and watching for blood pressure and heart rate changes that cause symptoms.

Time-Out: When the doctors, nurses, technologists, and all personnel that are participating in a surgery stop what they are doing (before the patient is sedated) and identify the patient, procedure being performed (including site of implant), technique to be used, and any other important patient information (such as drug allergies).

Transient Ischemic Attack (TIA): see Stroke.

Transvenous defibrillator: Most common type of defibrillator that uses leads placed through veins and attached to the heart.

Tricuspid valve: One-way valve that blood crosses when traveling from the right atrium to the right ventricle.

Twiddling: Manipulation of defibrillator or leads that may lead to malfunction.

Undersensing: Failure of a defibrillator to detect native heart signals that can lead to inappropriate pacing or failure to shock a potentially life-threatening arrhythmia.

Valvular cardiomyopathy: Heart failure caused by valve disease.

Vegetation: Collection of bacteria forming a mass that adheres to the defibrillator wires or inside of the heart.

Vena cava: Inferior and superior vena cava are the main vessels that return the body's blood to the right atrium.

Venography: X-ray of the veins taken after contrast is injected to assess if a pacemaker lead can be inserted.

<u>Ventricle, Left or Right</u>: Main pumping chambers that pump blood to the lungs and rest of the body.

<u>Voltage</u>: Electrical charge that can be measured or emitted by a defibrillator.

<u>Wand</u>: Small device placed on the chest over the defibrillator and connected by a wire to the programmer; the wand enables the defibrillator to communicate with the programmer.

<u>X-ray</u>: Special type of radiation used in medicine that is used to image bones and soft tissue.

References

Ahmed, I., E. Gertner, W. B. Nelson, C. M. House, R. Dahiya, C. P. Anderson, D. G. Benditt, and D. W. Zhu. 2010. "Continuing Warfarin Therapy Is Superior to Interrupting Warfarin with or without Bridging Anticoagulation Therapy in Patients Undergoing Pacemaker and Defibrillator Implantation." *Heart Rhythm* 7 (6): 745–49.

Alt, E., R. Volker, and H. Blomer. 1987. "Lead Fracture in Pacemaker Patients." *Thoracic Cardiovascular Surgery* 35: 101–4.

Alter P., S. Waldhans, E. Plachta, R. Moosdorf, and W. Grimm. 2005. "Complications of Implantable Cardioverter Defibrillator Therapy in 440 Consecutive Patients." *Pacing and Clinical Electrophysiology* 28: 926–32.

Bardy, G. H., K. L. Lee, D. B. Mark, J. E. Poole, D. L. Packer, R. Boineau, M. Domanski, C. Troutman,

J. Anderson, G. Johnson, S. E. McNulty, N. Clapp-Channing, L. D. Davidson-Ray, E. S. Fraulo, D. P. Fishbein, R. M. Luceri, and J. H. Ip, for the Sudden Cardiac Death in Heart Failure Trial (SCD-HeFT) Investigators. 2005. "Amiodarone or an Implantable Cardioverter-Defibrillator for Congestive Heart Failure." *The New England Journal of Medicine* 352 (3): 225–37.

Bayliss C. E., D. S. Beanlands, and R. J. Baird. 1968. "The Pacemaker-Twiddler's Syndrome: A New Complication of Implantable Transvenous Pacemakers." *Canadian Medical Association Journal* 99: 371–73.

Belott, P. "How to Access the Axillary Vein." 2006. *Heart Rhythm* 3 (3): 366–69.

Bohm, A., A. Pinter, and I. Preda. 2002. "Ventricular Tachycardia Induced by a Pacemaker Lead." *Acta Cardiologica* 57 (1): 23–24.

Bracke, F., A. Meijer, and B. Van Gelder. 2003. "Venous Occlusion of the Access Vein in Patients Referred for Lead Extraction: Influence of Patient and Lead Characteristics." *Pacing and Clinical Electrophysiology* 26: 1649–52.

Bristow, M. R., L. A. Saxon, J. Boehmer, S. Krueger, D. A. Kass, T. De Marco, P. Carson, L. DiCarlo, D. DeMets, B. G. White, D. W. DeVries, and A. M. Feldman, for the Comparison of Medical Therapy, Pacing, and Defibrillation in Heart Failure (COMPANION) Investigators. 2004. "Cardiac-Resynchronization Therapy with or without an Implantable Defibrillator in Advanced Chronic Heart Failure." *The New England Journal of Medicine* 350 (21): 2140–50.

Brockow, K., C. Christiansen, G. Kanny, O. Clément, A. Barbaud, A. Bircher, P. Dewachter, J. L. Guéant, R. M. Rodriguez Guéant, C. Mouton-Faivre, J. Ring, A. Romano, J. Sainte-Laudy, P. Demoly, W. J. Pichler, ENDA, and the EAACI Interest Group on Drug Hypersensitivity. 2005. "Management of Hypersensitivity Reactions to Iodinated Contrast Media." *Allergy* 60: 150–58.

Burns J. L., E. R. Serber, S. Keim, and S. Sears. 2005. "Measuring Patient Acceptance of Implantable Cardiac Device Therapy: Initial Psychometric Investigation of the Florida Patient Acceptance Survey." *Journal of Cardiovascular Electrophysiology* 16 (4): 384–90.

Cappato, R., H. Calkins, S. Chen, W. Davies, Y. Iesaka, J. Kalman, Y. Kim, G. Klein, A. Natale, D. Packer, A. Skanes. 2009. "Prevalence and Causes of Fatal Outcome in Catheter Ablation of Atrial Fibrillation." *Journal of the American College of Cardiology* 53 (19): 1798–803.

Carlson, M. D., and B. L. Wilkoff. 2006. "Recommendation from the HRS Task Force on Device

Performance Policies and Guidelines." *Heart Rhythm* 3: 1250–73.

Chadha T. S., and M. A. Cohn. 1983. "Noninvasive Treatment of Pneumothorax with Oxygen Inhalation." *Respiration* 44 (2): 147–52.

Cheng, A., Y. Wang, J. P. Curtis, and P. D. Varosy. 2010. "Acute Lead Dislodgements and In-Hospital Mortality in Patients Enrolled in the National Cardiovascular Data Registry Implantable Cardioverter Defibrillator Registry." *Journal of the American College of Cardiology* 56: 1651–56.

Cherubini, A., J. Oristrell, X. Pla, C. Ruggiero, R. Ferretti, G. Diestre, A. M. Clarfield, P. Crome, C. Hertogh, V. Lesauskaite, G. I. Prada, K. Szczerbinska, E. Topinkova, J. Sinclair-Cohen, D. Edbrooke, and G. H. Mills. 2011. "The Persistent Exclusion of Older Patients from Ongoing Clinical Trials Regarding Heart Failure." *Archives of Internal Medicine* 171 (6): 550–56.

Crilley, J. G., B. Herd, C. S. Khurana, C. A. Appleby, M. A. de Belder, A. Davies, and J. A. Hall. 1997. "Permanent cardiac pacing in elderly patients with recurrent falls, dizziness and syncope, and a hypersensitive cardioinhibitory reflex." *Postgraduate Medical Journal* 73: 415–18.

Curtis, A. B., S. J. Worley, P. B. Adamson, E. S. Chung, I. Niazi, L. Sherfesee, T. Shinn, and M. Sutton, for the Biventricular versus Right Ventricular Pacing in Heart Failure Patients with Atrioventricular Block (BLOCK HF) Trial Investigators. 2013. "Biventricular Pacing for Atrioventricular Block and Systolic Dysfunction." *The New England Journal of Medicine* 368: 1585–93.

Curtis, J. P., J. J. Luebbert, Y. Wang, S. S. Rathore, J. Chen, P. A. Heidenreich, S. C. Hammill, R. I. Lampert, H. M. Krumholz. 2009. "Association of Physician Certification and Outcomes among Patients Receiving an Implantable Cardioverter-Defibrillator." *The Journal of the American Medical Association* 301 (16): 1661–70.

DaCosta, S. S., N. A. Scalabrini, A. Costa, J. G. Caldas, and F. M. Martinelli. 2002. "Incidence and Risk Factors of Upper Extremity Deep Vein Lesions after Permanent Transvenous Pacemaker Implant: A 6-Month Follow-Up Prospective Study." *Pacing and Clinical Electrophysiology* 25: 1301–1306.

Datta, G., A. Sarkar, and A. Haque. 2011. "An Uncommon Ventricular Tachycardia due to Inactive PPM Lead." *ISRN Cardiology* Article ID 232648, 3 pages.

DiBiase, L., S. Conti, P. Mohanty, R. Bai, J. Sanchez, D. Walton, A. John, P. Santangeli, C. S. Elayi, S. Beheiry, G. J. Gallinghouse, S. Mohanty, R. Horton, S. Bailey, J. D. Burkhardt, and A. Natale. 2011. "General Anesthesia Reduces the

Prevalence of Pulmonary Vein Reconnection during Repeat Ablation when Compared with Conscious Sedation: Results from a Randomized Study." *Heart Rhythm* 8: 368–72.

Dimsdale, C., A. Dimsdale, J. Ford, J. B. Shea, and S. F. Sears. 2012. "My Child Needs or Has an Implantable Defibrillator: What Should I Do?" *Circulation* 126: e244–47.

D'Ivernois, C., J. Lesage, and P. Blanc. 2008. "Where Are Left Ventricular Leads Really Implanted? A Study of 90 Consecutive Patients." *Pacing and Clinical Electrophysiology* 31 (5): 554–59.

Ellenbogen, K. A., A. S. Hellkamp, B. L. Wilkoff, J. L. Camunas, L. C. Love, T. A. Hadjis, K. L. Lee, G. A. Lamas. 2003. "Complications Arising After Implantation of DDD Pacemakers: The MOST Experience." *American Journal of Cardiology* 92: 740–41.

Ellenbogen, K. A., M. A. Wood, D. M. Gilligan, M. Zmijewski, D. Mans, and the CAPSURE Z Investigators. 1999. "Steroid Eluting High Impedance Pacing Leads Decrease Short and Long-Term Current Drain: Results from a Multicenter Clinical Trial." *Pacing and Clinical Electrophysiology* 22 (1): 39–48.

Ellery, S. M., and V. E. Paul. 2004. "Complications of Biventricular Pacing." *European Heart Journal Supplements* 6 (Su D): D117–21.

Epstein, A.E., J. P. DiMarco, K. A. Ellenbogen, N. A. Estes, III, R. A. Freedman, L. S. Gettes, A. M. Gillinov, G. Gregoratos, S. C. Hammill, D. L. Hayes, M. A. Hlatky, L. K. Newby, R. L. Page, M. H. Schoenfeld, M. J. Silka, L. W. Stevenson, M. O. Sweeney, S. C. Smith, Jr., A. K. Jacobs, C. D. Adams, J. L. Anderson, C. E. Buller, M. A. Creager, S. M. Ettinger, D. P. Faxon, J. L. Halperin, L. F. Hiratzka, S. A. Hunt, H. M. Krumholz, F. G. Kushner, B. W. Lytle, R. A. Nishimura, J. P. Ornato, R. L. Page, B. Riegel, L. G. Tarkington, C. W. Yancy, American College of Cardiology/American Heart Association Task Force on Practice Guidelines (Writing Committee to Revise the ACC/AHA/NASPE 2002 Guideline Update for Implantation of Cardiac Pacemakers and Antiarrhythmia Devices), American Association for Thoracic Surgery, and Society of Thoracic Surgeons. 2008. "ACC/AHA/HRS 2008 Guidelines for Device-Based Therapy of Cardiac Rhythm Abnormalities A Report of the American College of Cardiology/American Heart Association Task Force on Practice Guidelines (Writing Committee to Revise the ACC/AHA/NASPE 2002 Guideline Update for Implantation of Cardiac Pacemakers and Antiarrhythmia Devices)." *Journal of the American College of Cardiology* 51 (21): e1–62.

Ezekowitz, J. A., B. H. Rowe, D. M. Dryden, N. Hooton, B. Vandermeer, C. Spooner, and F. A. McAlister. 2007. "Systematic Review: Implantable Cardioverter Defibrillators for Adults with Left Ventricular Systolic Dysfunction." *Annals of Internal Medicine* 147: 252–62.

Ezekowitz, J. A., P. W. Armstrong, and F. A. McAlister. 2003. "Implantable Cardioverter Defibrillators in Primary and Secondary Prevention: A Systematic Review of Randomized, Controlled Trials." *Annals of Internal Medicine* 138 (6): 445–52.

Faber, T. S., R. Gradinger, S. Treusch, C. Morkel, J. Brachmann, C. Bode, and M. Zehender. 2007. "Incidence of Ventricular Tachyarrhythmias during Permanent Pacemaker Therapy in Low-Risk Patients Results from the German Multicentre EVENTS Study." *European Heart Journal* 28 (18): 2238–42.

Fahraeus T., and C. J. Hoijer. 2003. "Early Pacemaker Twiddler Syndrome." *Europace* 5: 279–81.

Farling, P. A. 2000. "Thyroid Disease." *British Journal of Anaesthesia* 85 (1): 15–28.

Ferguson Jr., T. B., C. L. Ferguson, K. Crites, and P. Crimmins-Reda. 1996. "The Additional Hospital Costs Generated in the Management of Complications of Pacemaker and Defibrillator Implantations." *The Journal of Thoracic and Cardiovascular Surgery* 111: 742–52.

Fortescue, E. B., C. L. Berul, F. Cecchin, E. P. Walsh, J. K. Triedman, and M. E. Alexander. 2005. "Comparison of Modern Steroid-Eluting Epicardial and Thin Transvenous Pacemaker Leads in Pediatric and Congenital Heart Disease Patients." *Journal of Interventional Cardiac Electrophysiology* 14 (1): 27–36.

Freedman, A., M. T. Rothman, and J. W. Mason. 1982. "Recurrent Ventricular Tachycardia Induced by an Atrial Synchronous Ventricular-Inhibited Pacemaker." *Pacing and Clinical Electrophysiology* 5 (4): 490–94.

Fung, J. W., J. Y. Chan, R. Omar, A. Hussin, Q. Zhang, G. Yip, K. H. Lam, F. Fang, and C. M. Yu. 2007. "The Pacing to Avoid Cardiac Enlargement (PACE) Trial: Clinical Background, Rationale, Design, and Implementation." *Journal of Cardiovascular Electrophysiology* 18: 735–39.

Fyke, III, F. E. 1993. "Infraclavicular Lead Failure: Tarnish on a Golden Route." *Pacing and Clinical Electrophysiology* 16: 373–76.

Gaitan, B. D., T. L. Trentman, S. L. Fassett, J. T. Mueller, and G. T. Altemose. 2011. "Sedation and Analgesia in the Cardiac Electrophysiology Laboratory: A National Survey of Electrophysiologists Investigating the Who, How, and Why?" *Journal of Cardiothoracic and Vascular Anesthesia* 25: 647–59.

Germano, J. J., Reynolds, M., Essebag, V., Josephson, M.E. 2006. "Frequency and Causes of Implantable Cardioverter-defibrillator Therapies: Is Device Therapy Proarrhythmic?" *American Journal of Cardiology* 97: 1255–61.

Geyfman, V., R. H. Storm, S. C. Lico, and J. W. Oren, IV. 2007. "Cardiac Tamponade as Complication of Active-Fixation Atrial Lead Perforations: Proposed Mechanism and Management Algorithm." *Pacing and Clinical Electrophysiology* 30: 498–501.

Goldenberg, I, A. J. Moss, W. J. Hall, S. McNitt, W. Zareba, M. L. Andrews, and D. S. Cannom. 2006. "Causes and Consequences of Heart Failure after Prophylactic Implantation of a Defibrillator in the Multicenter Automatic Defibrillator Implantation Trial II." *Circulation* 113: 2810–16.

Gould, P. A. 2008. "Outcome of Advisory ICD replacement: One Year Follow-up." *Heart Rhythm* 5 (12): 1675–81.

Grammes, J. A., C. M. Schulze, M. Al-Bataineh, G. A. Yesenosky, C. S. Saari, M. J. Vrabel, J. Horrow,

M. Chowdhury, J. M. Fontaine, and S. P. Kutalek. 2010. "Percutaneous Pacemaker and Implantable Cardioverter-Defibrillator Lead Extraction in 100 Patients with Intracardiac Vegetations Defined by Transesophageal Echocardiogram." *Journal of the American College of Cardiology* 55 (9): 886–94.

Groeneveld, P. W., M. A. Matta, J. J. Suh, F. Yang, and J. A. Shea. 2007. "Quality of Life among Implantable Cardioverter-Defibrillator Recipients in the Primary Prevention Therapeutic Era." *Pacing and Clinical Electrophysiology* 30: 463–71.

Hampton, J. R., M. J. F. Harrison, J. R. A. Mitchell, J. F. Prichard, and C. Seymour. 1975. "Relative Contributions of History-Taking, Physical Examination, and Laboratory Investigation to Diagnosis and Management of Medical Outpatients." *British Medical Journal* 2: 486–89.

Hargreaves, M. R., A. Doulalas, and O. J. M. Ormerod. 1995. "Early Complications Following Dual Chamber Pacemaker Implantation: 10-Year Experience of a Regional Pacing Centre." *Eur JCPE* 5 (3): 133–38.

Hayes, D. L., and R. E. Vlietstra. 1993. "Pacemaker Malfunction." *Annals of Internal Medicine* 119 (8): 828–35.

Hirschl, D. A., V. R. Jain, H. Spindola-Franco, J. N. Gross, and L. B. Haramati. 2007. "Prevalence and Characterization of Asymptomatic Pacemaker and ICD Lead Perforation on CT." *Pacing and Clinical Electrophysiology* 30: 28–32.

Hunt, S. A., D. W. Baker, M. H. Chin, M. P. Cinquegrani, A. M. Feldman, G. S. Francis, T. G. Ganiats, S. Goldstein, G. Gregoratos, M. L. Jessup, R. J. Noble, M. Packer, M. A. Silver, L. W. Stevenson, R. J. Gibbons, E. M. Antman, J. S. Alpert, D. P. Faxon, V. F. A. K. Jacobs, L. F. Hiratzka, R. O. Russell, and S. C. Smith. 2001. "ACC/AHA Guidelines for the Evaluation and Management of Chronic Heart Failure in the Adult: Executive Summary A Report of the American College of Cardiology/American Heart Association Task Force on Practice Guidelines (Committee to Revise the 1995 Guidelines for the Evaluation and Management of Heart Failure)." *Circulation* 104: 2996–3007.

Iesaka, Y., T. Pinakatt, A. J. Gosselin, and J. W. Lister. 1982. "Bradycardia Dependent Ventricular Tachycardia Facilitated by Myopotential Inhibition of a VVI Pacemaker," *Pacing and Clinical Electrophysiology* 5 (1: 23–29.

Johansen, J. B., O. D. Jørgensen, M. Møller, P. Arnsbo, P. T. Mortensen, and J. C. Nielsen. 2011. "Infection after Pacemaker Implantation: Infection Rates and Risk Factors Associated with Infection in a Population-Based Cohort Study of 46299

Consecutive Patients." *European Heart Journal* 32 (8): 991–98.

Jordaens, L., E. Robbens, E. Van Wassenhove, and D. L. Clement. 1989. "Incidence of Arrhythmias after Atrial or Dual-Chamber Pacemaker Implantation." *European Heart Journal* 10 (2): 102–7.

Kikkenborg Berg, S., P. Moons, A.-D. Zwisler, P. Winkel, B. D. Pederson, P. Ulrich Pederson, and J. Hastrup Svendsen. 2013. "Phantom Shocks in Patients with Implantable Cardioverter Defibrillator: Results from a Randomized Rehabilitation Trial (COPE-ICD)." *Europace* 15 (10): 1463–67.

Klug, D., M. Balde, D. Pavin, F. Hidden-Lucet, J. Clementy, N. Sadoul, J. L. Rey, G. Lande, A. Lazarus, J. Victor, C. Barnay, B. Grandbastien, S. Kacet, and PEOPLE Study Group. 2007. "Risk Factors Related to Infections of Implanted Pacemakers and Cardioverter-Defibrillators." *Circulation* 116: 1349–55.

Knight, B. P., A. Desai, J. Coman, M. Faddis, and P. Yong. 2004. "Long-Term Retention of Cardiac Resynchronization Therapy." *Journal of the American College of Cardiology* 44 (1): 72–77.

Korte, T., H. Koditz, T. Paul, and J. Tebbenjohanns. 2004. "High incidence of appropriate and inappropriate ICD therapies in children and adolescents with implantable cardioverter defibrillator." *Pacing and Clinical Electrophysiology* 27 (7): 924–32.

Kulvatunyou, N., A. Vijayasekaran, A. Hansen, J. L. Wynne, T. O'Keeffe, R. S. Friese, B. Joseph, A. Tang, and P. Rhee. 2011. "Two-Year Experience of Using Pigtail Catheters to Treat Traumatic Pneumothorax: A Changing Trend." *Journal of Trauma* 71 (5): 1104–7.

Lawrence, V. A., S. G. Hilsenbeck, C. D. Mulrow, R. Dhanda, J. Sapp, and C. P. Page. 1995. "Incidence and Hospital Stay for Cardiac and Pulmonary Complications after Abdominal Surgery." *Journal of General Internal Medicine* 10: 671–78.

Lee, D. S., A. D. Krahn, J. S. Healey, D. Birnie, E. Crystal, P. Dorian, C. S. Simpson, Y. Khaykin, D. Cameron, A. Janmohamed, R. Yee, P. C. Austin, Z. Chen, J. Hardy, and J. V. Tu. 2010. "Evaluation of Early Complications Related to De Novo Cardioverter Implantation." *Journal of the American College of Cardiology* 55 (8): 774–82.

Lauer, M. S., G. S. Francis, P. M. Okin, F. J. Pashkow, C. F. Snader, and T. H. Marwick. 1999. "Impaired Chronotropic Response to Exercise Stress Testing as a Predictor of Mortality." *Journal of the American Medical Association* 281: 524–29.

Lemon J., S. Edelman, and A. Kirkness. 2004. "Avoidance behaviors in patients with implantable cardioverter defibrillators." *Heart & Lung* 33 (3): 176–82.

Leon, A. R., W. T. Abraham, A. B. Curtis, J. P. Daubert, W. G. Fisher, J. Gurley, D. L. Hayes, R. Lieberman, S. Petersen-Stejskal, K. Wheelan, MIRACLE Study Program. 2005. "Safety of Transvenous Cardiac Resynchronization System Implantation in Patients with Chronic Heart Failure: Combined Results of Over 2000 Patients from a Multicenter Study Program." *Journal of the American College of Cardiology* 46 (12): 2348–56.

Li, W., B. Sarubbi, and J. Somerville. 2000. "Iatrogenic Ventricular Tachycardia from Endocardial Pacemaker Late after Repair of Tetralogy of Fallot." *Pacing and Clinical Electrophysiology* 23 (12): 2131–34.

Link, M. S., N. A. M. Estes, J. J. Griffin, P. J. Wang, J. D. Maloney, J. B. Kirchhoffer, G. F. Mitchell, J. Orav, L. Goldman, G. A. Lamas. 1998. "Complications of Dual Chamber Pacemaker Implantation in the Elderly." *Journal of Interventional Cardiac Electrophysiology* 2: 175–79.

Lukl, J., V. Doupal, E. Sovová, and L. Lubena. 1999. "Incidence and Significance of Chronotropic Incompetence in Patients with Indications for Primary Pacemaker Implantation or Pacemaker Replacement." *Pacing and Clinical Electrophysiology* 22 (9): 1284–91.

Magney, J. E., D. M. Flynn, J. A. Parsons, D. H. Staplin, M. V. Chin-Purcell, S. Milstein, and D. W. Hunter. 1993. "Anatomical Mechanisms Explaining Damage to Pacemaker Leads, Defibrillator Leads, and Failure of Central Venous Catheters Adjacent to the Sternoclavicular Joint." *Pacing and Clinical Electrophysiology* 16: 445–47.

Magnusson, L., and D. R. Spahn. 2003. "New Concepts of Atelectasis during General Anesthesia." *British Journal of Anaesthesia* 91 (1): 61–72.

Mahapatra, S., K. A. Bybee, T. J. Bunch, R. E. Espinosa, L. J. Sinak, M. D. McGoon, D. L. Hayes. 2005. "Incidence and Predictors of Cardiac Perforation after Permanent Pacemaker Implantation." *Heart Rhythm* 2: 907–11.

Marcos, S. K., and H. S. Thomsen. 2001. "Prevention of General Reactions to Contrast Media: A Consensus Report and Guidelines." *European Radiology* 11 (9): 1720–28.

Mond, H. G., and A. Proclemer. 2011. "The 11th World Survey of Cardiac Pacing and Implantable Cardioverter-defibrillators: Calendar Year 2009—A World Society of Arrhythmia's Project." *Pacing and Clinical Electrophysiology* 34 (8): 1013–27.

Moss, A. J., W. J. Hall, D. S. Cannom, H. Klein, M. W. Brown, J. P. Daubert, N. A. Estes, E. Foster,

H. Greenberg, S. L. Higgins, M. A. Pfeffer, S. D. Solomon, D. Wilber, and W. Zareba. 2009. "Cardiac-Resynchronization Therapy for the Prevention of Heart-Failure Events." *The New England Journal of Medicine* 361(14): 1329–38.

Murkin, J. M. 1982. "Anesthesia and Hypothyroidism: A Review of Thyroxine Physiology, Pharmacology, and Anesthetic Implications." *Anesthesia & Analgesia* 61 (4): 371–83.

Nery, P. B., R. Fernandes, G. M. Nair, G. L. Sumner, C. S. Ribas, S. M. Menon, X. Wang, A. D. Krahn, C. A. Morillo, S. J. Connolly, and J. S. Healey. 2010. "Device-Related Infection among Patients with Pacemakers and Implantable Defibrillators: Incidence, Risk Factors, and Consequences." *Journal of Cardiovascular Electrophysiology* 21 (7): 786–90.

Noseworthy, P. A., I. Lashevsky, P. Dorian, M. Greene, S. Cvitkovic, and D. Newman. 2004. "Feasibility of Implantable Cardioverter Defibrillator Use in Elderly Patients: A Case Series of Octogenarians." *Pacing and Clinical Electrophysiology* 27: 373–78.

Oginosawa, Y., H. Abe, and Y. Nakashima. 2002. "The Incidence and Risk Factors for Venous Obstruction after Implantation of Transvenous Pacing Leads." *Pacing and Clinical Electrophysiology* 25: 1605–11.

O'Mahony, D. 1995. "Pathophysiology of Carotid Sinus Hypersensitivity in Elderly Patients." *Lancet* 346: 950–52.

Ong, J. J. C., P. C. Hsu, L. Lin, A. Yu, R. M. Kass, C. T. Peter, and C. D. Swerdlow. 1995. "Arrhythmias after Cardioverter-defibrillator Implantation: Comparison of Epicardial and Transvenous systems." *American Journal of Cardiology* 75 (2): 137–40.

Parsonnet, V., A. D. Bernstein, and B. Lindsay. 1989. "Pacemaker-Implantation Complication Rates: An Analysis of Some Contributing Factors." *Journal of the American College of Cardiology* 13 (4): 917–21.

Pedersen, S. S., K. C. van den Broek, R. A. M. Erdman, L. Jordaens, and D. A. M. J. Theuns. 2010. "Pre-implantation implantable cardioverter defibrillator concerns and Type D personality increase the risk of mortality in patients with an implantable cardioverter defibrillator." *Europace* 12: 1446–52.

Pedersen, S. S., S. F. Sears, M. M. Burg, and K. C. van den Broek. 2009. "Does ICD Indication Affect Quality of Life and Levels of Distress?" *Pacing and Clinical Electrophysiology* 32: 153–56.

Prudente, L. A., J. Reigle, C. Bourguignon, D. E. Haines, and J. P. DiMarco. 2006. "Psychological indices and phantom shocks in patients with ICD." *Journal of Interventional Cardiac Electrophysiology* 15: 185–90.

Reynolds, M. R., D. J. Cohen, A. D. Kugelmass, P. P. Brown, E. R. Becker, S. D. Culler, and A. W. Simon. 2006. "The Frequency and Incremental Cost of Major Complications Among Medicare Beneficiaries Receiving Implantable Cardioverter-Defibrillators." *Journal of the American College of Cardiology* 47 (12): 2493–97.

The Royal College of Radiologists. 2010. *Standards for Intravascular Contrast Administration to Adult Patients: Second Edition.* London: The Royal College of Radiologists.

Rozmus, G., J. P. Daubert, D. T. Huang, S. Rosero, B. Hall, and C. Francis. 2005. "Venous Thrombosis and Stenosis after Implantation of Pacemakers and Defibrillators." *Journal of Interventional Cardiac Electrophysiology* 13: 9–19.

Schulza, N., K. Puschelb, and E. E. Turkc. 2009. "Fatal Complications of Pacemaker and Implantable Cardioverter Defibrillator Implantation: Medical Malpractice?" *Interactive Cardiovascular and Thoracic Surgery* 8: 444–48.

Sears, S. F., and J. B. Conti. 2002. "Quality of Life and Psychological Functioning of ICD Patients." *Heart* 87: 488–93.

Sears, S. F., J. B. Shea, J. B. Conti. 2005. "How to Respond to an Implantable Cardioverter-Defibrillator Shock." *Circulation* 111: e380–82.

Sohail, M. R., S. Hussain, K. Y. Le, C. Dib, C. M. Lohse, P. A. Friedman, D. L. Hayes, D. Z. Uslan, W. R. Wilson, J. M. Steckelberg, L. M. Baddour, and Mayo Cardiovascular Infections Study Group. 2011. "Risk Factors Associated with Early- versus Late-Onset Implantable Cardioverter-Defibrillator Infections." *Journal of Interventional Cardiac Electrophysiology* 31(2): 171–83.

Stevenson, R., D. Lugg, R. Gray, D. Hollis, M. Stoner, and J. L. Williams. 2012. "Pacemaker Implantation in the Extreme Elderly." *Journal of Interventional Cardiac Electrophysiology* 33 (1): 51–58.

Tarakji, K. G., E. J. Chan, D. J. Cantillon, A. L. Doonan, T. Hu, S. Schmitt, T. G. Fraser, A. Kim, S. M. Gordon, B. L. Wilkoff. 2010. "Cardiac Implantable Electronic Device Infections: Presentation, Management, and Patient Outcomes." *Heart Rhythm* 7 (8): 1043–47.

Tramer, M. R., E. von Elm, P. Loubeyre, and C. Hauser. 2006. "Pharmacologic Prevention of Serious Anaphylactic Reactions Due to Iodinated Contrast Material: Systematic Review." *The BMJ* 333: 675–78.

Trcka, J., C. Schmidt, C. S. Seitz, E. B. Brocker, G. E. Gross, and A. Trautman. 2008. "Anaphylaxis to Iodinated Contrast Materials: Nonallergic Hypersensitivity or IgE-Mediated Allergy? *AJR* 190 (3): 666–70.

Trentman, T. L., S. L. Fassett, J. T. Mueller, and G. T. Altemose. 2009. "Airway Interventions in the Cardiac Electrophysiology Laboratory: A Retrospective Review." *Journal of Cardiothoracic and Vascular Anesthesia* 23: 841–45.

van den Broek, K. C., M. Habibovic, and S. S. Pedersen. 2010. "Emotional Distress in Partners of Patients with an Implantable Cardioverter Defibrillator: A Systematic Review and Recommendations for Future Research." *Pacing and Clinical Electrophysiology* 33: 1442–50.

van Rees J. B., M. K. de Bie, J. Thijssen, C. J. W. Borleffs, M. J. Schalij, and L. van Erven. 2011. "Implantation-Related Complications of Implantable Cardioverter-Defibrillators and Cardiac Resynchronization Therapy Devices." *Journal of the American College of Cardiology* 58 (10): 995–1000.

van Rooden, C. J., S. G. Molhoek, F. R. Rosendaal, M. J. Schalij, A. E. Meinders, and M. V. Huisman. 2004. "Incidence and Risk Factors of Early Venous Thrombosis Associated with Permanent

Pacemaker Leads." *Journal of Cardiovascular Electrophysiology* 15: 1258–62.

Wang, N. C., J. L. Williams, S. K. Jain, and A. Shalaby. 2009. "Post-Pacemaker Pulsations." *American Journal of Medicine* 122: 345–47.

Wiegand, U. K. H., D. LeJeune, F. Boguschewski, H. Bonnemeier, F. Eberhardt, H. Schunkert, and F. Bode. "Pocket Hematoma After Pacemaker or Implantable Cardioverter Defibrillator Surgery: Influence of Patient Morbidity, Operation Strategy, and Perioperative Antiplatelet/Anticoagulation Therapy." *CHEST* 126 (4): 1177–86.

Wilkoff, B. L. 2007. "How to Treat and Identify Device Infections." *Heart Rhythm* 4: 1467–70.

Williams, J. L., D. Lugg, R. Gray, D. Hollis, M. Stoner, and R. Stevenson. 2010. "Patient Demographics, Complications, and Hospital Utilization in 250 Consecutive Device Implants of a New Community Hospital Electrophysiology Program." *American Heart Hospital Journal* 8 (1): 33–39.

Williams, J. L., and R. T. Stevenson. 2012. *Complications of Pacemaker Implantation, Current Issues and Recent Advances in Pacemaker Therapy*. Edited by Attila Roka. http://www.intechopen.com/books/current-issues-and-recent-advances-in-pacemaker-therapy/complications_of_pacemaker_implantation.

Williams, J. L., V. Valencia, D. Lugg, R. Gray, D. Hollis, J. W. Toth, R. Benson, M. DeFranceso-Loukas, R. T. Stevenson, and P. J. Teiken. 2011. "High Frequency Jet Ventilation During Ablation of Supraventricular and Ventricular Arrhythmias: Efficacy, Patient Tolerance and Safety." *The Journal of Innovations in Cardiac Rhythm Management* 2: 1–7.

Worley, S. J., D. C. Gohn, R. W. Pulliam, M. A. Raifsnider, B. Ebersole, and J. Tuzi. "Subclavian Venoplasty by the Implanting Physicians in 373 Patients over 11 Years." *Heart Rhythm* 8 (4): 526–33.

Writing Committee to Revise the ACC/AHA/NASPE 2002 Guideline Update for Implantation of Cardiac Pacemakers and Antiarrhythmia Devices. 2008. "ACC/AHA/HRS 2008 Guidelines for Device-Based Therapy of Cardiac Rhythm Abnormalities A Report of the American College of Cardiology/ American Heart Association Task Force on Practice Guidelines." *Journal of the American College of Cardiology* 51 (21): e1–62.

Yu, C. M., J. Y. S. Chan, Q. Zhang, R. Omar, G. W. K. Yip, A. Hussin, F. Fang, K. H. Lam, H. C. K. Chan, and J. W. H. Fung. 2009. "Biventricular Pacing in Patients with Bradycardia and Normal Ejection Fraction." *The New England Journal of Medicine* 361 (22): 2123–34.

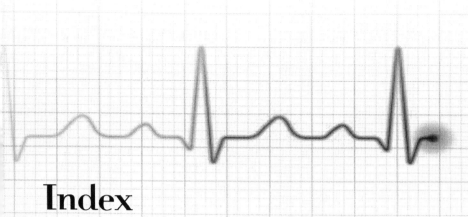

Index

About the Author

Jeffrey L. Williams, MD, is board certified in internal medicine, cardiovascular disease, and clinical cardiac electrophysiology and is currently medical director of electrophysiology at the Good Samaritan Hospital. He double majored in biomedical and electrical engineering at Vanderbilt University and then obtained his master's degree in bioengineering from the University of Pittsburgh, where he was awarded a Keck Fellowship for graduate school. Earning his medical degree from Drexel University in Philadelphia, Dr. Williams then went on to complete five years of fellowship training in both cardiovascular disease and clinical cardiac electrophysiology at the University of Pittsburgh Medical Center. Possessing extensive knowledge and a unique background in both engineering and cardiology, Williams has earned numerous accolades within academic and clinical settings, including awards from both the American College of Cardiology Foundation and the National Institutes of Health. Dr. Williams directs the only community-hospital-based Heart Rhythm Center in the United States that published outcomes for pacemaker and defibrillator implantations. He was elected Governor of the Pennsylvania Chapter of the American College of Cardiology (2016-2019).

Made in the USA
Columbia, SC
29 April 2017